St. Francis Nursing Center
2 Ridgewood Parkway
Newport News, VA 23602

REVISED
SOCIAL SERVICE CARE PLANS
FOR LONG TERM CARE FACILITIES

by
Marylou Hughes, LCSW, DPA
Manuela Espinosa

M & H Publishing Company, Inc.
P. O. Box 268
La Grange, Texas 78945-0268

Second Printing July 1989
Third Printing December, 1989
Fourth Printing May, 1990
Fifth Printing November, 1990
Sixth Printing May, 1991
Seventh Printing March 1992

ISBN: 1-877735-11-6

Copyright © 1989 by M & H Publishing Company, Inc.
All rights reserved. No part of this publication may be
reproduced, stored in a retrieval system or transmitted, in
any form or by any means, electronic, mechanical,
photocopying, recording or otherwise, without the prior
written permission of the publisher.

ABOUT THE AUTHORS

Dr. Marylou Hughes received her doctorate degree in Public Administration from Nova University in Fort Lauderdale, Florida, and has a Master of Social Work from the University of Utah in Salt Lake City, Utah. She has undergraduate majors in sociology and psychology. For the past twenty plus years she has worked in social services as an employee of the Department of Health and Rehabilitative Services in Florida, and later in rehabilitation and mental health centers and hospitals. She is currently self-employed as a marriage counselor, psychotherapist, teacher and consultant to several private facilities in Florida.

Dr. Hughes has also written *The Nursing Home and the Resident's Relatives*, 1987; *Enhancing the Self Esteem of the Nursing Home Resident*, 1987; and *Mental Health Problems and the Nursing Home Resident*, 1988.

Ms. Manuela Espinosa is a native of Ecuador but received her education from Pasadena City College in California. She has been an active member of her professional and civic organizations and has many years of experience as an activity director in long term care facilities and working with clients in the hospital. Her responsibilities included social care planning as the Social Service designee. She is presently employed in that capacity at Vero Beach Care Center in Vero Beach, Florida..

Marylou Hughes dedicates this book to
Araminta B. and John H. Hughes

Acknowledgements to:

Mary Cacciatore, who emphasizes the restorative approach

All examples are generalized from typical nursing home incidents, and are not reports of actual situations.

TABLE OF CONTENTS

SECTION I - CARE PLAN DEFINED

    CARE PLAN DEFINED 3
    THE BEGINNING 4
    SOCIAL SERVICE ASSESSMENT 9
    DISCHARGE PLANNING 17
    THE MIDDLE 24
    THE END 26

SECTION II - CARE PLAN EXAMPLES

    ADJUSTMENT 30

        Depression 30
        Hopelessness 31
        Terminal Illness 32
        Family Does Not Accept Prognosis 34
        Pain 35
        Cancer 35
        Desire to Die 37
        Will Not Accept Inability to Walk 38
        Stroke 38
        Feeling of Uselessness 39
        Suicidal 40
        Death of Loved One 41
        Nursing Home Adjustment 42
        Family Unhappy with Resident's Care 44
        Abusive Towards Disoriented Residents 45
        Loss of Hearing and Vision 46
        Incontinent 46
        Unsafe Smoking 47
        Fear of Loss of Ability 48
        Lack of Motivation 48
        Resident and Relative Do Not Accept
            Aging Process 49
        Cannot Express Self Verbally 50
        Lonely and Alone 50
        Apprehensive and Demanding Because of Fears   51
        Boredom 52
        Misses Animals 52

Wants Independence 53

BEHAVIOR

Anxiety 54
Disoriented 56
Mood Swings 57
Angry, Suspicious, Abusive 58
Dependent 60
Manipulative 61
Fear of Bath 62
Unresponsive 62
Refuses to See Doctor 63
Malnourished 63
Distractible 64
Delusions 65
Complaints About Physical Health 66
Wanders 66
Hallucinations 67

MATERIAL NEEDS

Special Treats 68
Special Aids 68
Exploitation 69
Short Term Placement 69
Finances Depleted 70
Transportation 70

RELATIONSHIPS

Infrequent Family Visits 72
Does Not Get Along With Roommate 72
Roommate Dies 73
Will Not Accept Roommate 74
Orders Roommate Around 74
Dominates Residents' Council 75
Younger Resident 76
No Relatives or Friends 77
Family Does Not Keep Promises 77
Need For Privacy 78

SECTION III - HELP FOR THE HELPER

QUARTERLY PROGRESS NOTES 83

PSYCHOSOCIAL APPROACHES 87

    Reality Orientation 87
    Validation 88
    Self-Esteem Enhancement 89
    Restorative Techniques 90
    Non-Verbal Communication 90
    Distraction 91
    Reassurance 91
    Participation 92
    Supportive 93
    Re-direct 93
    Listening 94
    Anticipation of Needs 95
    Behavior Modification 95
    Modeling 97
    Reminiscence 98

INVOLVING FAMILIES AND THE COMMUNITY 99

ORGANIZING THE JOB 101

AVOIDING BURN-OUT 105
    Reasons for Burn-Out 105
    Prevention of Burn-Out 107

RELAXATION 109

REMOTIVATION 111

RESOCIALIZATION 113

NURSING HOME VISITING TIPS 114

INDEX 117

SECTION I
CARE PLAN DEFINED

CARE PLAN DEFINED

If you have worked in a nursing home for longer than a week, you know by now that a care plan is something that must be done and that you are to be involved in doing it. You realize that paper work is frequent and that care plans are required! But, a care plan is more than just writing down something at a meeting with other nursing home professionals.

The care plan is the connective tissue for the entire staff of the nursing home. It represents the plan of action taken by each team member on the behalf of the resident. It is a statement of what the individual can expect over and above and along with the regular daily care he/she receives. The care plan tells the story of the resident's strengths and weaknesses, needs and problems, and how to achieve a change. There is a beginning, middle, and end.

The care plan format is uniformly as follows.

DATE PROBLEM/NEED GOAL APPROACH ASSIGNMENT DATE
    (strengths   RESOLVED
      to build on)

THE BEGINNING

A care plan is completed for each resident at the time he/she is admitted to the nursing home. Each member of the care team contributes to this plan. The team generally consists of:

1. Nursing Home Department Heads and/or representatives

    Director of Nursing
    Head Nurse
    Activities Director
    Social Service Director
    Head of Dietary Staff
    Nursing Aide Supervisor
    Physical Therapist
    Others (Housekeeping Department, Consultants,
        Administrator, Physician, Speech Therapist,
        Occupational Therapist, Maintenance Department)
    Pharmacist

2. Resident and Representatives

    Resident
    Resident's Family
    Friends
    Volunteers
    Clergy
    Social Service Agency Representatives
    Attorney
    Legal Guardian
    Significant Others (Roommate, Neighbor, Ombudsman)

The care plan for each resident is revised each quarter. The team will meet to discuss each resident on a regular basis depending on need and requirements, but at least every ninety days. There may be specially called care plan meetings because of:

1. Changes in the residents' health, behavior, family situation, or emotional status.

2. Skilled care requirements.

3. Staff needs for planning an unified approach to residents' problems.
4. Staff frustrations about how best to help the resident.
5. Family or resident dissatisfaction with care.

A master list of all residents with the scheduled time for care plan review should be made available to staff so that everyone knows when the care plan meeting will be held. Residents and families can also be made aware of the time so they can attend and be part of the planning.

Care plan meetings that have the best attendance meet at a special time, and this time is set aside and adhered to. In this way staff members from each discipline can plan their schedules. The residents and families will also know when to appear.

One staff member is designated to head the care plan meeting. It functions better if one person is responsible to see that meetings are held and an expected format is in place. It does not matter who is the leader, as long as it is a person who can organize the agenda, be available, give everyone a chance to contribute, acknowledge each person's contribution, and still keep the meeting moving.

Some topics to cover on each resident are:
1. Problems related to the medical diagnosis.
2. Problems with medications and why the resident is taking particular medications.
3. Patterns of behavior.
4. Areas where rehabilitation and restoration can be addressed.
5. Interpersonal difficulties.
6. Family relationships.
7. Areas of personal distress.
8. Who does what, i.e., assignment of responsibilities for tasks.

Assignments are usually made according to discipline responsibility and knowledge, but in many instances can be assigned to all or several disciplines. Examples of problems that need to be assigned to all staff are eating, communication, and adjustment difficulties, and inappropriate and unsafe behavior. On occasion there may not be a clear cut social service problem, but the social worker can contribute by assisting the resident in other areas where there are problems that cause unhappiness or maladjustment. Most problems encompass social, behavioral, physical, and emotional aspects. Who does what is not as important as that it is done. Although an approach may be assigned to the social worker, it can be carried out by a volunteer or a family member working under the auspices of the social service department. The fact that it is done is the crucial thing. How it was done is then documented.

Some care plans can continue indefinitely as the residents' problems continue. Instances of ongoing or intermittent depression need constant attention. The chronic depressives need to be motivated, encouraged to eat and care for themselves properly, be evaluated for medication, have people to invite them places, and projects to entice them. They need compassion and companionship and listening and caring. The residents with cyclical depressions need preventative approaches, plans for early warning and intervention when the first signs of depression are noted, and specialized help during the depression to make it less severe in depth and length.

Other ongoing problems are:

Terminal illness.
No support system.
Communication difficulties.
Mood swings.
Wandering.
Family maladjustments.
Sexual acting out
Problems related to specific diseases such as:
    Diabetics who will not follow diets.
    Anxiety in COPD.
    Impulsivity in stroke patients.
    Brain damaged who strike out at others.

Approaches may change as more effective methods are deterined. But do not change what is working.

Problems, goals, and approaches sometimes need to be abandoned as unrealistic, unworkable, or ineffective. When the same problem persists and the goals are not reached month after month, it is time for reevaluation and a change in goal and/or approach. If the problem remains there needs to be a new way to attack it. Maybe the wrong approach has been used or the wrong goal set. Maybe there has been progress, but it is not measurable. Emotions are seldom measurable, behavior are. The goal could be to decrease crying to one time a day instead of saying that the mood will be happier. It is easy to know when the behavior of crying stops. The emotion of a happier mood is not so easy to document.

There are many ways to measure goal achievement. The ability to count what has happened is perhaps the easiest. Measurable goals may be expressed as follows.

> The resident will wheel herself to the dining room three out of five times.
> The resident will attend activities two days a week.
> The resident will say hello to three people a day.
> The resident will be out of the room fifty percent of the day.
> The resident will agree to an eye examination within two weeks.
> The resident will not wander away from the facility for the next quarter.
> The resident will control his/her agitation during the morning hours.
> The resident will have his/her hair styled before the next review.
> The resident will leave the facility for an outing.
> The resident will go to the activity room one time a day.

A care plan recording form follows.

CARE PLAN

NAME: _____ AGE: _____ DATE ADMITTED: _____

PHYSICIAN: _____ DATE OF INITIAL CONFERENCE: _____

DIAGNOSIS: _____

DISCHARGE PLAN: _____

Key:
- A - Administration
- MD - Physician
- N - Nurse
- P - Pharmacist
- D - Dietary
- FM - Family
- SW - Social Worker
- ST - Speech Therapist
- OT - Occup. Therapist
- AT - Activities
- PT - Physical Therapist
- O - Other

DATE	PROB. NO.	PROBLEM/NEED	PROJ. DATE	GOALS	APPROACHES	Date Resolved or Changed	Assigned To	SIGNATURE

SOCIAL SERVICE ASSESSMENT

To prepare for the care plan meeting and to help devise a constructive plan for each resident the social worker completes a social service assessment. The assessment includes the following:

1. Social History

    a. Identifying information (Name, address, age, nickname, sex, marital status, education, race, nationality, finances, religion, occupation, reason for nursing home placement)

    b. Background information (History of relationships with, friends, family, employers, community organizations, adjustments to parenting, loss of spouse, health problems, retirement, living arrangements prior to nursing home placement)

2. Assessment of Current Functioning

    a. Resident's current relationship to family (Where does family live? What can family provide? How honest are they with resident? How often will they visit? How long have they lived together?)

    b. Resident's and family's feeling about nursing home placement (Who recommended nursing home placement? Is there blame, guilt, resentment or other negative emotions present? Is this a temporary or permanent arrangement? What are their expectations of nursing home staff? Are attitudes realistic?)

    c. Resident's reaction to current illness, handicap, or disability (Describe physical appearance, grooming, and clothes. Notice non-verbal communication such as posture, facial expression and body movements. Is the verbal communication lucid and sensible or unclear and rambling? Are there special emotional problems with depression, anger or mood? How has resident coped with any physical problems of seeing, hearing, speaking, walking, pain, or dependence?)

3. Identification of Social Service Needs

    a. Material needs (Finances, items for comfort, pleasure, or of necessity, legal services, medically prescribed equipment, transportation, special treats, or hobbies)

    b. Social needs (Special roommate requirements, relationships with family, friends, other nursing home residents, and staff, interests and preferences as to time place and type of activity)

    c. Emotional needs (Does resident prefer privacy or company? Does resident feel easily threatened, or is he/she welcoming to everyone? Is resident having difficulty adjusting to loss of spouse, home, independence, pets? Is resident in need of reassurance, security, and approval? How does resident handle sadness, anger, fear? What is resident's method of getting his/ her needs met?)

4. Plan to Meet Needs

    a. Problem/Need (The problem or need is identified. Is there something missing in this resident's life that the social worker can provide or arrange? Is there something in this person's life-style that is important to maintain and nurture for his/her continued happiness? What special strengths can be utilized and enhanced?)

    b. Goal (What is to be the final result after the problem/need is identified? What is to be accomplished that will enhance the quality of the resident's life?)

    c. Approach/Plan (What is the social worker going to do in order to obtain the goal?)

    d. Date expected to meet goal (Can the approach prove effective in one month, two months, three or four months?)

5. Discharge Plan

    a. Rehabilitation potential (Based on the resident's diagnosis, resources, and family support, is it good, poor, or is there no potential?)

    b. Plans for discharge (How does the resident, the staff, the family, view the discharge and what arrangements can be made for his/her continuity of care?)

c. Resources and referrals needed at discharge (What community resources, such as the Home Health Agency, the Council on Aging, Vocational Rehabilitation, or the Housing Authority will be needed to facilitate the discharge?)

A narrative social service assessment incorporating the information in the outline follows.

Social History

Ms. S. is an 80 year old widowed woman who was transferred to the nursing home from the local hospital where she underwent surgery to repair a broken left hip. She will remain in the nursing home for therapy and rehabilitation until she is able to return to her daughter's home.

Ms. S. was brought from Italy by her parents when she was three years old. They moved immediately to this area where she has lived ever since. She married before completing high school and was married for fifty two years before her husband died twelve years ago. She has not worked outside of the home. Her husband worked for the county road department. She lives on this pension plus social security. She is an avid Catholic and attends mass three or four times a week.

Ms. S. has never been a joiner and feels uncomfortable in large groups other than her family. She has been friends with her neighbors but devoted herself to caring for her home, her husband, and her children. She still grieves for the loss of this role and has never adjusted to her husband's death. She has always enjoyed housework and since moving in with her daughter, son-in-law, granddaughter, and great-granddaughter has found some satisfaction managing the household while everyone is at work. Four other children (and their families) live out of state.

Assessment of Current Functioning

Resident's family is eager to have her return to the home. They have come to depend on her, love her, and miss her. Since they live locally and the family is quite large they expect one family member will be able to visit each evening.

The family is accustomed to hearing Mrs. S. complain and meet her concerns with reassurance and half-truths.

Ms. S. is embarrassed and unhappy about being in the nursing home. Her family led her to believe that she was going to a rehabilitation center. She now doubts their word that this is a temporary arrangement and thinks that they are trying to get rid of her because she is old, no longer useful, and is loudly accusing them of throwing her away. She feels guilty that she may have done something wrong and keeps going over past experiences that she should have handled differently. Her family feels guilty because they feel they should be doing more for Ms. S. but cannot give her the amount of care she needs at this time in their own home. Their guilt sometimes turns to resentment that Mother wants more than they can provide. Ms. S. expects the nursing home staff to cure her immediately so that she can be worthwhile again. She refuses to participate in anything that might be fun because she wants to put all her time into getting well and useful. The family wants the nursing staff to make Mother happy. Since Mother is not happy and they feel helpless they come to the staff with every complaint the resident has, indicating that the staff is being neglectful.

Ms. S. wears a hearing aid, has had cataract operations, and wears glasses. She is alert, oriented in time, place, and person, and lucid in her thinking. She has been a healthy woman. Until recently she had been hospitalized only to give birth to her children and for a gall bladder operation many years ago. She has false teeth. She suffers from minor arthritis in her hands and feet and wonders if this clumsiness turned her family against her. She suspects that that is the reason she fell. She is depressed and wonders if she will ever be able to function on her own again. She dislikes having the staff care for her and apologizes whenever she needs them to do anything for her. She works well in physical therapy, but has derogatory comments about her own efforts.

Identification of Social Service Needs

Ms. S.'s family keeps her supplied with treats, clothes, and self-help equipment. They bring her everything they think will make her happier. Since she does not like the nursing home food, they have taken to bringing her a meal each evening.

Ms. S. is not a socializer. She is a doer. She needs to be involved in activities that make her feel she is helping herself or others. She likes calling the nurse for her roommate. She does her physical therapy exercises almost to excess. She has enjoyed the resident exercise group.

Ms. S. needs to know that her family does want her to return. She needs reassurance that through her own efforts she will be able to go home again. She also needs some help in understanding that her family loves her no matter what she can or cannot do, and that her being able to go home does not revolve around her being able to take complete responsibility for the household. Her family needs help in listening to her, really hearing her concerns, and responding to them, instead of just brushing them aside as they have been doing.

Plan to Meet Needs

This close family is not communicating well. Consequently, none of the family members is getting the reassurance they need.

The social worker will try to help the family understand what the resident needs to know and help the resident hear what the family is saying.

To accomplish this the social worker will stop and talk with the resident one time a day to let her express her feelings and fears and help her set up ways to achieve her goals. The social worker will be in constant contact with the family so that they do not unintentionally mislead the resident. The social worker will help them keep their anxiety within reasonable bounds. Both resident and family will be encouraged to attend a care plan conference so that they see the staff working together for the same goal, which is rehabilitation and discharge. This should be accomplished within three months.

Discharge Plan

When Ms. S. regains her mobility there is no reason she cannot be returned to her family's home. She should be able to manage there with a walker and continue her physical therapy on an out-patient basis through home health services. The priest at Ms. S.'s church will keep involved in the process as he has been a calming influence during the nursing home experience and can probably help Ms. S. adjust to a more limited role in the home.

General Information on Social Service Assessments

Social service assessments need not be long and tedious. Insomuch as the vital statistics and major problems and needs are reported, the assessment is a unique contribution. If it is too wordy, other busy, staff members will not want to take time to read it. And read it they should, because the social service assessment gives information about relationships in regard to facts, feelings, and patterns that is not available elsewhere.

Most nursing homes now use a Social Service Assessment form. This proves to be a time saver and a point of quick reference. It does not, however, give the picture of the resident as well as the narrative style does. If the assessment form is used the progress notes assume greater importance in conveying the essence of the resident's and the family's personality, attitudes, and interactions.

An example of social service assessment form is next.

ADMISSION AND SOCIAL INFORMATION   Today's Date _____

PERSONAL INFORMATION:

Admission Date: _____ From _____ Physician _____

Name: _____ Age: _____
    Last   First   Maiden or Middle

Home Address: _____
    Street   City   State   Zip   County

Date of Birth: _____ Place of Birth _____

Race: _____ Sex _____ Marital Status M ___ S ___ W ___ D ___ Citizen of what country? _____

Religion _____ Church Affiliation _____

Minister _____ Phone No. _____ Desire Visits? _____

Name of local funeral home desired: _____

Education: Elementary _____ High School _____ College _____ Other _____

Occupation: (Last Position) _____ Military Service _____

Financial Situation: (Monthly income) _____ Source: _____

Medicare # _____ Social Security # _____ Medicaid # _____

Responsible Party _____ Relationship _____

Address: _____ Phone No. _____

Occupation: _____ Place of Employment _____ Phone No. _____

MEDICAL INFORMATION: Diagnosis (es): _____
_____ Patient informed? Yes ____ No ____

Physician's Estimate of Restorative Potential _____

Physician's Address: _____ Phone No. _____

Dentist _____ Podiatrist _____ Other Dr.s _____

Discharge Plan _____

FAMILY AND SOCIAL INFORMATION: Pre-Admission Living Arrangements:

Father's Name: _____ Mother's Maiden Name _____

Lived alone _____ With Others _____ With Whom _____ House _____ Apt. _____

Address _____ Who Planned Placement? _____

Events Leading to Admission _____

Patient's Attitude toward placement? _____ Family's _____

FAMILY AND FRIENDS IMPORTANT TO PATIENT:

_____
Name   Relationship   Address   Phone

_____
Name   Relationship   Address   Phone

Adjustment
to Retirement: _____

Number of
Family Members: Sons ____   Daughters ____   Brothers ____   Sisters ____   Grandchildren ____
Great grandchildren ____ Other relatives ____ Pets - what kind _____

INTERESTS/ACTIVITIES:
                                    Present   **Past**   **Comments**

Music/Plays instrument? _____
Reading _____
Current events _____
Sports _____
Crafts _____
Reminiscing _____
Sewing/Needlework _____
Bingo _____
Poker/other card games _____
Exercise _____
Parties _____
Television programs _____
Movies/what kind _____
Other games _____
Clubs & Organizations _____
Will family provide materials for hobbies? _____
Interest in personal appearance? _____
Special talent/achievements _____
Most significant event of life _____
Travel experiences _____
People w/greatest influence on my life _____
Registered Voter? _____   Desires to Vote: Yes _____ No _____

CURRENT FUNCTIONING: COMMUNICATION _____

BEHAVIOR				**HABITS**		**AIDS**	
Quiet	____	Noisy	____	Nonsmoker	____	Eyeglasses	____
Friendly	____	Demanding	____	Smokes	____	Dentures	____
Alert	____	Depressed	____	Pipe	____	Hearing Aid	____
Anxious	____	Disoriented	____	Cigarettes	____	Prosthesis	____
Confused	____	Secure	____	Cigars	____	Crutches	____
Wanders	____	Seek Support	____	Chews tobacco	____	Walker	____
Walks alone	____	Other	____	Dips snuff	____	Cane	____
Feeds self	____			Drinks	____	Wheelchair	____
Dressing	____			Other	____	Brace	____
Bowel control	____					Pacemaker	____
Bladder	____					Colostomy	____
						Catheter	____

Sleeping Habits _____

DIETARY INFORMATION: Weight _____ **Height** _____
Favorite meal: Breakfast _____ Lunch _____ Dinner _____ Snacks _____ Favorite foods: _____
Problem foods: _____

                              Social Worker's Signature _____

DISCHARGE PLANNING

Discharge planning starts the day the resident enters the nursing home. The social worker begins collecting information regarding how the residents managed before nursing home placement and what resources will be available to them when they leave the nursing home. It is crucial to be knowledgeable about community resources and know how to obtain services for the residents upon their discharge to the least restrictive environment.

The discharge plan needs the specific contribution of each discipline with exact goals for what must be accomplished by the resident before a discharge occurs.

Community Resources

Most frequently used community resources follow.

Mental and Addiction Problems

>Alcoholics Anonymous
>Mental Health Center

Health Problems

>Bureau of the Blind
>Cancer Society
>Deborah Society
>Diabetes Foundation
>Hospice
>Hospital
>Health Department
>Medical Equipment Rentals
>Home Health Agency
>Ostomy Association
>Alzheimer Support Group
>Ambulance
>Reach for Recovery
>Stroke Club
>Rehabilitation Clinic

Home Delivered Services (Transportation, Respite Care), Housekeeping Services, Meals on Wheels, Shopping)

    Council on Aging

Financial Assistance

    Employment Service
    Food Stamps
    Social Security (Medicare, Medicaid)
    Red Cross
    Welfare Department
    Salvation Army
    Vocational Rehabilitation
    Veterans Administration

Housing

    Housing Authority
    Welfare Department
    Salvation Army

Placement on Discharge

Where may the residents go so that they will be serene and secure and still manage to obtain the needed care? Their choices are preeminent. Starting with the setting providing the most personal freedom, the choices include:

    Own home, living alone
    Own home with spouse
    Own home with relative
    Own home with hired live-in help
    Relative's home
    Supervised care in a licensed boarding home
    Foster Home
    Rehabilitation Center
    Hospital

Discharge Potential

The discharge potential is part of the social work assessment, the initial care plan, and each subsequent care plan. The discharge possibility may be:

    Excellent
    Good
    Fair

Marginal
Guarded
Poor
None

Discharge Limitations

Discharge is hindered by any number of emotional, physical, financial, and relationship problems. A discharge can be constrained because of one or more of the following.

Refusal of the resident to leave.
Psychological dependence.
Overprotection by relatives or staff.
Physical disability (sight, speech, hearing, ambulation, reaching, holding, etc.)
Psychiatric problems.
Twenty four hour supervision needed.
Total dependency in activities of daily living.
Continued deterioration.
Complicated medical regime.
Seizures.
Family refuses to care for resident.
Family cannot care for resident because of other responsibilities.
Restricted finances

This next form can be used in the social service progress notes. It indicates the up-to-date discharge plan.

LONG TERM GOAL AND DISCHARGE PLANNING
DISCHARGE CONSIDERATION

GOOD (50% chance of reaching potential)
POOR (Less than 50% change of reaching potential)
NONE (not at all realistic)

LONG TERM GOAL—DISCHARGE CONSIDERATION - DATE: _____

    GOOD _____ POOR _____ NONE _____

1. The patient will return to living with _____
   when rehabilitated of the problems which are _____
   _____ have been accomplished.
2. The patient is in the terminal stages of the disease process, which is _____ .
   Support services and skilled nursing care are required.
3. Skilled nursing care is required on a 24 hour basis for _____
   _____
4. Other _____

LONG TERM GOAL—DISCHARGE CONSIDERATION - DATE: _____

    GOOD _____ POOR _____ NONE _____

1. The patient will return to living with _____
   when rehabilitated of the problems which are _____
   _____ have been accomplished.
2. The patient is in the terminal stages of the disease process, which is _____ .
   Support services and skilled nursing care are required.
3. Skilled nursing care is required on a 24 hour basis for _____
   _____
4. Other _____

LONG TERM GOAL—DISCHARGE CONSIDERATION - DATE: _____

    GOOD _____ POOR _____ NONE _____

1. The patient will return to living with _____
   when rehabilitated of the problems which are _____
   _____ have been accomplished.
2. The patient is in the terminal stages of the disease process, which is _____ .
   Support services and skilled nursing care are required.
3. Skilled nursing care is required on a 24 hour basis for _____
   _____
4. Other _____

Patient's Name _____ Admission Date _____

Keeping track of referrals is not always easy and remembering to enter them into the residents' progress notes can slip the mind. The referral log is useful for staying current until quarterly up-dates are done.

SOCIAL SERVICE REFERRAL LOG

RESIDENT	Date	Alzheimer's Support Group	Transportation	Social Security	Rehabilitation	Optometrist	Mental Health	Material Needs	Legal Services	HRS	Hospice	Hospital	Home Health	Dentist	Consultant	Clergy	Alcoholics Anonymous	Other

There is now a picture of the residents' family, interests, former life-style, and way of coping with problems. There is good indication of how well the resident will relate to others and how helpful the family will be. There is some idea of whether this will be a short or long term nursing home placement. Based on the assessment, made with the help of information gathered by the other team members and from the resident and the family, you are ready to begin a plan of care for the individual.

You are prepared for the care plan meeting. You, the residents, and the nursing home team can make a constructive plan of care that will be geared to helping the residents and their significant others adjust to the trauma of nursing home placement. Your mutual plan will go beyond adjustment and acceptance to include enhancement. Nursing home living may be seen as a new way of life, with new satisfactions and opportunities. To accomplish this everyone needs to work together. To work together everyone has to know which way to go. The care plan gives that direction.

You have a good beginning. Now what?

THE MIDDLE

During the next three months you have the opportunity to evaluate your care plan. Is it workable? Is it effective? Does the resident respond positively to it? Does the family endorse it and cooperate?

Is the identified problem an agreed upon problem? If your assessment work was thorough, it will be. But sometimes our initial impressions will need revision. People change. We change. Problems change. There will be growth and there will be regression. Nothing stands still. Perhaps the problem is only a problem to the staff. For example, the resident may be content in what is perceived to be isolation. If this is the case, the identified problem is not the resident's. It is the staff's. If you, the social worker, see this, what do you do? You recognize that you are dealing with a dynamic situation. You are in the middle of the story. You do as any good writer would do. You document your new information. The progress note pages are there for you. You can give everyone the benefit of your observations and knowledge. As a social worker, only you have your particular perspective on the problem.

You get another chance at the goal. Does it look as though you will achieve the goal this quarter? If not, will it just take more time? Does it look as though the goal will never be achieved? Will you know when the goal is achieved? Can you verify that you have taken steps to reach the goal? Can you put in writing that these steps have either taken you nearer the goal or have had no or a negative effect?

If you are having trouble with the goal, you may have to take another look at it. Is it measurable? Will you know when you have accomplished what was wanted? Is it realistic? Can the residents honestly be expected to do what is wanted of them? Or does it require time, effort, and ability that you do not have? Is it specific? If the goal is measurable and reachable, it will probably be specific. We would not expect a goal for a resident to be happy to be either measurable or realistic. Neither is it specific. It is a lovely goal. But total, constant happiness is too much to expect of anyone. Is it realistic to expect the resident to be happy when the relatives visit? Maybe you would like to help the individual feel delight in a new accomplishment. Perhaps you would enjoy having the resident wake up happy. This is measurable and specific, but if the person has been a grump every morning of their eighty-three years, it is not a realistic goal.

The problem and the goal come before you decide on your approach. If we look at the goal of happiness we note that the approach would be different if we wanted to work with the residents on accomplishing new skills, enjoying their relatives, or being cheerful in the morning. The approach must be as realistic, as measurable, and as specific as your goal. Remember, you are documenting what you are doing. You cannot document what cannot be done. Are you going to help the resident be happy over a new skill by teaching and praising them four, seven, three, or two times a day, a week, a month? What is realistic? What can you do? How much help does the resident need for success?

Is it adequate that you are the only one involved in the approach? In order to achieve the goal do you need to enlist the help of nursing, dietary, activities, volunteers, or the family? This is part of your approach, part of the resident's permanent care plan, and part of your quarterly documentation in the resident's chart. Your planning and recording will represent the social work approach and will be consistent with what other specialties are doing to follow the care plan and deliver quality care to the nursing home resident.

THE END

What are the results? Was the approach carried out? If it was not, why not? Was the problem solved? Was the goal achieved? Did the residents find some satisfaction in this change or process? Were the relatives involved and helpful? How do we know the answers to all these questions? We know because you have written in the progress notes what you, the resident, and the significant others have done to contribute to the goal. You have told us what happened, why it happened, and how everyone felt about it. We have the results. The paper work is completed and so is the job — almost.

It is with a good story, as it is in life; the end is only the beginning of another chapter. The problem may be solved, may need more work, or may be unworkable. You can decide whether to continue to work on it, abandon it, or determine a new approach to solve it. Here is your chance to do it all over again and write a new ending!

SECTION II
CARE PLAN EXAMPLES

CARE PLAN EXAMPLES

To use this book it is necessary to know the residents and adapt the ideas for care plans to them. The examples are not designed to go directly from the book to the residents' care plan, but to give a broad outline of what is possible in the way of constructive care plans for those living in long term care facilities.

There is more satisfaction in doing care plans if the problem is narrowed from the general emotion, condition, or situation to a specific behavior or incident. Working on the specific brings results and a sense of accomplishment. Progress and effectiveness can be seen.

The care plans in the examples should be brought into even more focus to concentrate on single symptoms and applied to the behavior of the residents. It is possible to measure behaviors. Emotions can only be judged.

Remember that what follows are only examples. What is presented is a series of typical problems, possible goals, and approaches to stimulate your imagination and thinking. They can be reworded, rephrased, and applied to meet the needs of the residents with whom you are working. The approaches are suggestions for meeting the goals. Adjust the approaches to your residents, your work style, and your resources.

ADJUSTMENT

Example

Ms. A is terminally ill. She is depressed and feels hopeless. The family is not accepting the prognosis and wants her to get well.

PROBLEM/NEED: (Depression)

1. Resident refusing food.
2. Resident cries frequently.
3. Resident withdrawing from social contacts.
4. Resident complains of unhappiness.

GOAL:

1. Resident will attend one group activity a day.
2. Resident will attend therapeutic exercise class five days per week.
3. Resident will reminisce one time a day to see the value in her life.
4. Resident will discuss sad feelings and fears with professional staff by (date).
5. Resident will understand her grief by (date).
6. Resident will be evaluated by a psychiatrist by (date).
7. Residant will understand diagnosis by (date).
8. Resident will learn of her importance to others by (date).
9. Resident will learn to live one day at a time by identifying one pleasurable occurrence each day.
10. Resident will eat seventy-five percent of all offered food.

APPROACH:

1. Staff will determine resident's likes, dislikes, and interests.
2. Resident will be assisted to attend the activity of her choice on a daily basis.
3. Resident will be taken to exercise class by (staff, volunteer).
4. Staff member will see resident daily to discuss important events and memories of her past life.

5. Resident will have weekly appointments with social worker to work through fears and feelings regarding prognosis.
6. Appointment will be made with psychiatrist by (date).
7. Doctor, R.N., and other professional staff will discuss the facts of the resident's diagnosis and prognosis with her.
8. Staff members will tell resident of her contribution to them and to others one time each day.
9. Resident will be reminded of the pleasure of the present by staff pointing out an interesting or noteworthy event one time a day.
10. Resident will be offered foods she likes and snacks between meals.
11. Resident will be seated with companionable people in the dining room.

PROBLEM/NEED: **(Hopelessness)**

1. Resident shows no interest in activities.
2. Resident refuses to get out of bed.
3. Resident sees no reason to live.
4. Resident withdraws from social contacts.
5. Resident not interested in how she looks.

GOAL:

1. Resident will identify one interest by (date).
2. Resident will eat in the dining room one time a day.
3. Resident will understand that her life has meaning to others by (date) through identifying two things she has contributed to the lives of (others, her children, staff, friends).
4. Resident will accept a daily visit from the volunteer.
5. Resident will select her clothes each day.
6. Resident will go to the beauty parlor weekly.

APPROACH:

1. Staff will determine residents' likes and dislikes.
2. Staff will offer resident different activities to interest her.
3. Staff will tell resident of her strong points and how she brings pleasure to them and others.
4. Staff will help family let the resident know what her life means to them.
5. Volunteer will visit daily at a regularly scheduled time.
6. Nursing assistant will help resident decide on clothes for the day by giving her choices.
7. Beauty parlor appointments will be made.
8. Resident will be complimented and praised for good grooming.

PROBLEM/NEED: (Terminal illness)

1. Resident does not accept diagnosis.
2. Resident is taking out anger on staff members.
3. Resident is fearful of dying.
4. Resident wants to get affairs in order.
5. Resident worried that she may not have funds to pay for funeral.

GOAL:

1. Resident will discuss diagnosis with (doctor, R.N., social worker, family) by (date).
2. Resident will see that her anger is misplaced by (date) by stating what makes her angry.
3. Resident will understand that anger is a normal reaction to her diagnosis by (date).
4. Resident will channel anger away from staff and towards the disease by (date).
5. Resident will discuss her fears of dying with (doctor, R.N., social worker, family) by (date).
6. Resident will express anger appropriately one time a day.

7. Resident will make wishes known regarding funeral arrangements by (date).
8. Resident will make will by (date).
9. Resident will review funds and make payment arrangements for funeral by (date).

APPROACH:

1. (Doctor, nurse, social worker, family) will mention diagnosis to resident one time a day to make it real to her and desensitize her to it.
2. Staff, family will accept resident's handling of information regarding diagnosis, be it anger, depression, bargaining, denial, hopelessness, or acceptance.
3. Resident will be seen by a professional psychotherapist by (date).
4. Staff and family will learn to not take resident's anger personally.
5. Resident will have weekly scheduled sessions with the psychotherapist.
6. Resident will be visited by a funeral director by (date).
7. Resident will be seen by an attorney for the writing of her will and handling of her estate by (date).
8. Resident will be helped to name a person to carry out her final wishes by (date).
9. Resident will discuss her ideas about death by (date) with (professional).
10. Appointment will be made for resident to see clergy of her choice by (date).
11. Resident will be kept occupied on a daily basis with activities of her choice.
12. Resident will be visited daily by (staff, family, volunteer).
13. Funds will be set aside to pay for her funeral.

PROBLEM/NEED: (Family does not accept prognosis)

1. Resident upset because family will not let her speak of her fears of death.
2. Resident refusing to see her family.
3. Resident criticizes family when they visit.

GOAL:

1. Resident will have one successful visit with family by (date).
2. Resident will agree to see one family member by (date).
3. Resident will be able to talk to one family member about her impending death by (date).
4. Resident will formulate one positive thought about family by (date).
5. Resident will understand family's denial of her terminal illness by (date).
6. Resident will accept family members for what they can do for her by (date).

APPROACH:

1. Social worker will discuss resident's needs to talk about her fear with family by (date).
2. Social worker will help family understand their denial by (date).
3. Social worker will engage family in role playing to help them understand resident by (date).
4. Social worker will explain family's actions to resident by (date).
5. Social worker will work with resident to list positive aspects of her family by (date).
6. Social worker will assist resident in selecting one family member she can talk with by (date).
7. Family and resident will be seen together by a professional to explore mutual fears by (date).
8. Resident will have people other than her family with whom she can express her misgivings.

Example

Mr. B is in pain from cancer. He states that he would like to die.

PROBLEM/NEED: (Pain)

1. Resident demands increasing amounts of pain medications.
2. Resident refuses activities, complaining of pain.
3. Resident is withdrawing from others because of pain.

GOAL:

1. Resident will have needed medications for pain control.
2. Resident will learn relaxation to alleviate own pain by (date).
3. Resident will tolerate one activity every other day.
4. Resident will see one visitor a day.

APPROACH:

1. Resident will have a medical consultation regarding pain medication.
2. Pain medication will be evaluated on a bi-weekly basis to determine if it is meeting pain control needs.
3. Resident will discuss medications and effects and be one of the team members in evaluating how best to medicate for pain.
4. Resident will be offered different activities until one is found that does not aggravate his pain.
5. (Volunteer, family member, social worker) will visit daily.
6. Social worker will teach resident relaxation techniques by (date) and continue to relax with resident one time a week.
7. Resident will be provided with soothing music on a daily basis.

PROBLEM/NEED: (Cancer)

1. Resident has many questions regarding diagnosis.
2. Resident will not discuss diagnosis.
3. Resident denies diagnosis.
4. Resident claims he has the flu.

5. Resident wants to see another doctor.
6. Resident cannot discuss health problems with family as they brush off concerns by telling him he will soon be well.

GOAL:
1. Resident will have health questions answered by (date).
2. Resident will see physician of his choice by (date).
3. Resident will have his wishes regarding discussion of disease respected by all staff immediately.
4. Resident's family will learn to listen to him by (date).
5. Resident will keep up his hope as evidenced by one hopeful statement a day.

APPROACH:
1. (Social worker, M.D., nurse) will schedule daily time to answer resident's questions.
2. Resident will not be forced to discuss diagnosis, but staff will not enter into conspiracy of silence and will discuss diagnosis naturally and non-threateningly as health problems arise.
3. (Social worker, nurse, family) will make appointment for second opinion by (date).
4. Staff will accept resident's denial, but will continue to use appropriate terminology about cancer and not agree or disagree with resident.
5. Social worker will model appropriate health discussion with resident to family by (date).
6. Social worker will discuss family's fear regarding diagnosis with them by (date).
7. Social worker will be available to hear resident express his concern regarding disease's progression on a weekly basis.
8. Information regarding the disease will not be forced on the resident.
9. All expressions of hope from the resident or the family will be accepted.

PROBLEM/NEED: (Desire to die)

1. Resident refuses medications.
2. Resident refuses to eat.
3. Resident states he wants to die.
4. Resident will not get out of bed.
5. Resident exhibits no interest in (family, activities, events).
6. Resident threatens to kill self.

GOAL:

1. Resident will complete "Living Will" by (date).
2. Resident will drink liquid nourishment and fluids daily.
3. Resident will do what he can do for himself each day.
4. Resident will review his life one time each week.
5. Resident will reminisce daily.
6. Resident will have family support by (date) in the form of (daily visits, acceptance of diagnosis, expression of caring).
7. Resident will not harm self.

APPROACH:

1. (Social worker, family) will explain provisions of "Living Will" to resident. He will be helped to complete "Living Will" if this is his desire.
2. Fluids and liquid nourishment will be offered resident all day long by each staff member as they enter the room, or on an hourly basis (whichever is most frequent).
3. (Social worker, nurse, nursing assistant, activities) will assist resident to do what he can do for himself. He will be offered equipment for washing, eating, grooming, and given choices on schedule, clothing, activity, and food selection.
4. Social worker will meet with resident each week to review life's disappointments, accomplishments, and events.
5. (Social worker, family, nursing assistant, nurse, activities) will encourage resident to reminisce about life on a daily basis.

6. Social worker will encourage key family members to visit daily just to be with resident and provide comfort and support.
7. Resident will be kept under constant supervision.
8. All objects that can be used for self-harm will be removed from resident's area.

Example

Ms. C cannot accept inability to walk as a result of a stroke. She feels useless and expresses a wish to kill herself.

PROBLEM/NEED: (Will not accept inability to walk)

1. Resident refuses to work during physical therapy.
2. Resident sees using a wheelchair as failure.

GOAL:

1. Resident will work during physical therapy one time a week.
2. Resident will use wheelchair to propel self to dining room one time a week.

APPROACH:

1. Resident will be taken to physical therapy three times a week.
2. Staff will use behavior modification techniques with resident, praising and rewarding all efforts.
3. Advantages of using a wheelchair will be pointed out to resident one time a day.

PROBLEM/NEED (Stroke)

1. Resident cannot accept self with limitations.
2. Resident is embarrassed by disability.
3. Resident refuses to be with others because of altered self-image.

GOAL:

1. Resident will see one aspect of self that has not changed by (date).
2. Resident will learn that she is accepted by others in spite of her handicap by (date).
3. Resident will attend one spectator event each week.

APPROACH:

1. Staff will point out one aspect of resident that remains unchanged (looks, hair, verbal ability, friends, family, compassion, friendliness) one time a day.
2. (Staff, family, volunteers) will let resident know that she is liked and appreciated one time a day.
3. Resident will be taken to performances, exhibitions, movies, and other group spectator events one time a week.

PROBLEM/NEED: (Feeling of uselessness)

1. Resident feels she cannot do anything.
2. Resident is not doing what she can do.
3. Resident's self-esteem is based on her ability to be physically active.

GOAL:

1. Resident will do one thing to help someone else by (date).
2. Resident will do one thing to help herself by (date).
3. Resident will identify three good qualities about herself by (date).
4. Resident will have an opportunity to explore feelings with a mental health specialist by (date).

APPROACH:

1. Resident will be assigned a meaningful task by (date).

    Examples of meaningful tasks follow:

Be a foster grandparent	Feed pets
Change calendars	Water plants
Write thank you letters	Take group attendance
Serve on committees	Join resident council
Join RSVP	Make bed
Sort clothes	Stuff envelopes
Sell tickets	Arrange flowers
Help at sales	Write newsletter
Clerical work	Decorate for special events
Make name tags for doorways	

Work on dining room seating arrangements
   Help other residents through visits, reading, writing

2. Resident will take charge of her own (grooming, dressing, writing, telephoning) by (date).

3. Staff will praise resident for each attempt and each success.

4. (Staff, family, volunteers) will tell resident of the important role she has in the life of others, i.e., friend, member of a group or organization, neighbor, mother, wife, grandmother, sister.

5. Resident will be evaluated by a mental health specialist by (date).

6. (Staff, family, volunteer) will point out resident's abilities and qualities to her.

PROBLEM/NEED: (Suicidal)

1. Resident talks about killing herself.

2. Resident states she would rather be dead.

3. Resident makes statements that indicate that she does not plan to be around long, i.e. "When this is all over" or "I won't be a bother much longer."

GOAL:

1. Resident will not kill self.

2. Resident will recognize one reason for living by (date).

3. Resident will discuss concerns with mental health professional by (date).

APPROACH:

1. Staff will supervise resident constantly.

2. Staff will be available to listen to resident's concern on a daily basis.

3. Mental health professional will evaluate and treat resident by (date).

4. Social worker will explore feelings with resident through twice weekly appointments.

5. (Family, volunteer, staff) will take resident on outings to her favorite places.
6. Resident will be helped to be involved with one activity per day.
7. Resident will be introduced to potential friends.

Example

Mr. D's wife died. After her death there was no one to care for him in his home. He had to go to live in a nursing home. He complains about being in a nursing home to his children and makes them feel guilty. They are visiting less, for shorter periods of time, and blaming the staff for their father's discontent.

PROBLEM/NEED: (Death of a loved one)

1. Resident states that life has no meaning without his wife.
2. Resident cannot sleep at night.
3. Resident complains of overwhelming fatigue.
4. Resident has exacerbation of chronic health problem/arthritis.
5. Resident continues to talk to wife.
6. Resident states he feels wife's presence and fears he may be going crazy.

GOAL:

1. Resident will identify one reason to live by (date).
2. Resident will be able to relax and rest at night by (date).
3. Resident will participate in exercise program daily.
4. Resident will be up and out of room fifty percent of the day light hours.
5. Resident will understand the symptoms of grief by (date).
6. Resident will meet one new person every week.
7. Resident will find relief from arthritic symptoms in one month.
8. Resident will verbally work on his grief on a daily basis.
9. Resident will know he is not going crazy by (date).

APPROACH:

1. Resident will be invited to attend weekly reminiscence group.
2. Resident's talents and interests will be evaluated.
3. Resident will be offered activities he has enjoyed in the past.
4. (Staff, family, friends) will point out resident's value on a daily basis.
5. Resident will attend relaxation group.
6. Resident will be taught to relax by self in his room.
7. Staff will learn what resident's nighttime routine has been and help him carry this out in the nursing home.
8. Resident will be provided a calm and comforting nightly routine (warm milk, soft music, quiet room, back rub).
9. Social worker will let resident know the normal symptoms of grief, i.e., fatigue, loss of self-esteem, exacerbation of chronic health problems, sense of presence of lost loved one, sleeplessness, poor appetite, lack of concentration and interest, and assure him that he is not going crazy.
10. Resident will be invited and helped to daily exercise program.
11. Resident will be taken to meals outside of his room, to activity program, on outings with family and with other nursing home residents.
12. Resident will participate in resocialization program.
13. Resident's arthritis will be evaluated by M.D. and comfort measures will be introduced.
14. (Staff, family, friends) will listen to resident tell the story of his wife's death.

PROBLEM/NEED: (Nursing home adjustment)

1. Resident complains about being in a nursing home.
2. Resident blames family for nursing home placement.
3. Resident states he will not stay in the nursing home.
4. Resident tries to get family to remove him from nursing home.

5. Resident tries to leave nursing home.

GOAL:

1. Resident will be specific about two of his complaints about nursing home care so that staff can meet needs by (date).
2. Resident will discuss two reasons why family cannot care for him by (date).
3. Resident will state one reason why he needs nursing home care by (date).
4. Resident will express one benefit of nursing home care by (date).
5. Resident will have one visit a month with family without pressuring for removal from the nursing home.
6. Resident will continue to have family visits one time a week.
7. Resident will leave nursing home only on scheduled outings.

APPROACH:

1. Staff will listen to resident's complaints without getting defensive.
2. Staff will help resident focus his complaints about the nursing home on tangible difficulties that can be remedied.
3. Staff will make any feasible change in response to resident's complaints.
4. Social worker will listen to complaints about family and help him understand (a) family's contributions to him, (b) his own needs for care, (c) why family cannot care for him.
5. Staff will help resident see the benefits of nursing home care, i.e., twenty-four hour care, medication supervision, medical care, nutritional food, companionship, activities, attention to individual needs.
6. Social worker will help family understand resident's need for their support and caring through weekly contacts with them.
7. Social worker will help family handle their guilt through weekly contacts with them.
8. Social worker will help resident make better use of family visits.

9. Staff will monitor family visits, documenting frequency and length of time of each one.
10. (Family, staff) will arrange frequent outings for resident.
11. Staff will supervise resident carefully to prevent elopements.

PROBLEM/NEED: (Family unhappy with resident's care)

1. Resident not getting the benefit of family's visits as they spend most of the time complaining to the staff.
2. Resident not maintaining positive relationships with family as he uses the time for griping.

GOAL:

1. Resident will learn two ways to make family visits more rewarding by (date).
2. Resident will receive major proportion of family visit time by the end of the month.

APPROACH:

1. Staff will help resident learn to share events from his present life with family through reminding him of interesting happenings and activities and giving him information to tell family and encouraging him to bring up humorous incidents and memories of past and present life. This will help to refocus his topics of conversation for family visits.
2. Social worker will help family refocus visits by giving them a list of visiting tips.
3. Family will be asked to write down complaints and hand them to a specific staff member.
4. Family will be urged to make an appointment with (staff member) to air complaints so it will not interfere with visiting times.
5. Staff will make every effort to respond to all complaints within forty-eight hours.

Example

Ms. E needs assistance with her activities of daily living. She is alert and oriented and does not tolerate the residents who are not. She is rude, critical, and bossy to the disoriented.

PROBLEM/NEED: (Abusive toward disoriented residents)

1. Resident refuses to leave her room as she does not want to associate with disoriented residents.
2. Resident openly criticizes disoriented residents. Two have tried to physically hurt her in retaliation.
3. Resident is insulting to disoriented residents, upsetting them and others who overhear her.

GOAL:

1. Resident will understand she cannot change the disoriented resident by (date).
2. Resident will be kept occupied in her room and with other oriented, alert residents by (date).
3. Resident will be involved in volunteer program by (date).

APPROACH:

1. Process of aging and intellectual deterioration in certain diagnoses will be explained to resident and likened to her physical deterioration.
2. Staff will make it clear to resident that she is not responsible for monitoring the behavior of other residents.
3. Social worker will explore resident's fears regarding her own aging process, her feelings about living with those less intellectually capable than she is, and help her come to terms with her own adjustment through weekly and as needed interviews.
4. Resident will be assigned special projects.
5. Resident will help select own compatible roommate.
6. Resident will join activity group for alert, oriented residents.
7. Resident will be asked to volunteer with the Retired Senior Volunteer Program and assigned work to her liking.

Example

Mr. F does not hear or see well, but denies any problem. He blames any failing on others' poor speech habits or bad lighting. Thus, it is difficult to talk to him or set up a system of communication.

PROBLEM/NEED: (Loss of hearing and vision)

1. Resident complains that others do not speak up.
2. Resident complains about the poor lighting in the facility.
3. Resident complains about the television reception.

GOAL:

1. Resident will have a hearing evaluation by (date).
2. Resident will have eyes tested by (date).
3. Resident will understand non-verbal communication by (date).

APPROACH:

1. Appointment will be made with audiologist by (date).
2. Appointment will be made with ophthalmologist by (date).
3. Family will be informed of examinations and asked to help with the plan.
4. Staff will use body language to reinforce spoken word.
5. Staff will move close, speak clearly, make sure resident sees lips.
6. Staff will reinforce any gains resident makes in communication skills through praise and attention.

Example

Ms. G is incontinent of urine, but denies it and hides her dirty laundry.

PROBLEM/NEED: (Incontinent)

1. Resident is embarrassed by incontinence.
2. Resident gets hostile with anyone who brings up subject of urine incontinence.
3. Resident hides dirty laundry.
4. Resident tries to wash out sheets in the bathroom.

GOAL:

1. Resident will go to the bathroom at scheduled times to prevent accidents.

2. Resident will be evaluated for a catheter by (date).
3. Resident will put laundry in soiled laundry cart one time a day.

APPROACH:

1. Bladder training will be instigated.
2. When it is necessary to discuss incontinence with resident it will be done in a private place in a nonjudgmental way.
3. The benefits of a catheter will be discussed with the resident by (date).
4. Resident will be asked to place and be praised for placing laundry in soiled laundry cart on a daily basis.
5. Staff member will check resident and room at regular intervals.

Example

Mr. H is a long time heavy smoker. Although medically contraindicated his doctor no longer orders that he cannot smoke as he begged cigarettes from others and stole cigarette butts from ash trays. Mr. H smokes in non-smoking areas, burns his clothes with ashes, and starts fires in wastebaskets with his discarded cigarette butts.

PROBLEM-NEED: **(Unsafe smoking)**

1. Resident smokes in no smoking areas.
2. Resident burns clothes with cigarette ashes.
3. Resident starts fires in waste baskets.

GOAL:

1. Resident will smoke in designated areas only.
2. Resident will smoke only with supervision.
3. Resident will obtain cigarettes from (staff member).

APPROACH:

1. Family and friends will be asked to give all cigarettes for resident to (staff member).
2. Resident will be escorted to smoking area whenever he wants to smoke, as often as necessary.

3. Resident will obtain cigarettes from (staff member).
4. Resident's smoking will be supervised by (staff member).
5. Resident will have designated, supervised, smoking times.

Example

Ms. I fears deterioration, at times is overcome by these worries, and is unmotivated to do anything. Her daughter gets caught up in the resident's fears and becomes unrealistic about the aging process.

PROBLEM/NEED: (Fear of loss of ability)

1. Resident cannot enjoy present because of fear of the future.
2. Resident focuses on potential losses.
3. Resident worries about loss of (eye sight, orientation, physical ability, hearing).

GOAL:

1. Resident will focus on one present pleasure by (date).
2. Resident will learn one method for refocusing worries by (date).
3. Resident will see one way that she has already compensated for her limitations by (date).

APPROACH:

1. Resident will be helped to pick what she enjoys doing and have that pleasure reinforced on a daily basis.
2. Resident will be taught one method for refocusing worries (self-reassurance, thought replacement, focusing on facts, relaxation, meditation). Staff member will practice method with her two times per week.
3. Resident will be helped to see how she has already adjusted to and compensated for limitations and has continued to contribute and enjoy life.

PROBLEM/NEED: (Lack of motivation)

1. Resident wants others to do everything for her.
2. Resident does not want to do what she can do.

3. Resident neglects her (hair, make-up, friends, correspondence, attendance at events, family, activities, clothes).

GOAL:

1. Resident will make two decisions a day regarding her (schedule, clothes, activities).
2. Resident will (wash own face, comb own hair, write one letter, take self to dining room, call a friend) each day.

APPROACH:

1. Resident will be offered choices by (nursing assistant, nurse, social worker, activities) at least two times per day.
2. (Social worker, activities, nurse, nursing assistant) will assist and encourage resident in self-help procedures daily.

PROBLEM/NEED: **(Resident and relative do not accept aging process)**

1. Resident sees daughter's concern and her own fears escalate.
2. Resident feels daughter will no longer be pleased with her if she deteriorates.
3. Daughter raises resident's expectations that normal aging processes can be changed or reversed.

GOAL:

1. Resident and daughter will read material regarding diagnosis, prognosis, and normal aging process by (date).
2. Resident and daughter will attend family council meeting on (date) when speaker will discuss aging process.
3. Resident and daughter will attend meeting of (Alzheimer's group, stroke, ostomy, diabetes club) by (date).
4. Resident will learn to see daughter's concerns as caring about her rather than as a pressure to never change by (date).
5. Resident and daughter will discuss mutual problem with social worker by (date).
6. Resident and daughter will be aware of problem by (date).

APPROACH;

1. Reading material will be given to resident and daughter by (date) and discussed with them by (date).
2. Resident and daughter will be invited to family council meeting.
3. Resident and daughter will be told of health organization's meeting and urged to attend.
4. Resident and daughter will meet with social worker to become aware of and discuss problem and look for solutions by (date).

Example

Mr. J cannot make himself understood through verbalization. He appears lonely and tends to isolate himself.

PROBLEM/NEED: (Cannot express self verbally)

1. Resident cannot express self verbally and has not developed any non-verbal means of communication.

GOAL:

1. Resident will have speech evaluation by (date).
2. Resident will learn to nod yes or no by (date).
3. Resident will make eye contact by (date).
4. Resident will indicate desires by hand gestures by (date).
5. Resident will have a communication board by (date).

APPROACH:

1. Schedule speech evaluation by (date).
2. Work with resident daily so he will indicate yes or no with a nod.
3. Look in resident's eyes when talking with him.
4. Work with resident daily on appropriate hand signals.
5. Talk with family about purchasing a communication board for the resident.

PROBLEM/NEED: (Lonely and alone)

1. Resident seems happier with one to one contact.

2. Resident has not made friends.
3. Resident gets agitated in group activities.
4. Visitors do not spend much time with resident.

GOAL:

1. Resident will learn to smile at others by (date).
2. Resident will have one visitor every day.
3. Resident will meet one other person with whom he can spend time by (date).
4. Resident will respond to hugs by (date) with (smiles, return hugs, any indication of pleasure).

APPROACH:

1. One smile will be coaxed from the resident each day. He will be rewarded with a hug and extra time spent with him.
2. Family, volunteers, social worker will visit each day for fifteen minutes.
3. Resident will start in resocialization program on (date).

Example

Ms. K has lung problems and frequent episodes of shortness of breath. Because of her fears regarding this she is apprehensive and demanding.

PROBLEM/NEED: (Apprehensive and demanding because of fears regarding shortness of breath)

1. Resident refuses to go on outings.
2. Resident demands attention immediately.
3. Resident fears any change.

GOAL:

1. Resident will go on one outing a month.
2. Resident will get immediate attention for her shortness of breath.
3. Resident will have preparation for and accept one minor change a month.

APPROACH:

1. Resident will be scheduled for outings that are short in duration, close to the facility, in good weather, and when accompanied by a nursing assistant with whom she feels secure.
2. Resident will be helped immediately when medically necessary and at all times will be approached calmly and confidently. She will be shown concern and caring. Serene behavior will be modeled for her.
3. Changes will be avoided. When they are necessary she will be told at the optimum time so she will not develop anxiety. All her questions will be answered and her concerns alleviated.

Example

Mr. L had an active life and is at loose ends in the nursing home. He is bored and misses his animals.

PROBLEM/NEED: (Boredom)

1. Resident complains that days are long and uninteresting.

GOAL:

1. Resident will have a regular schedule to keep every day.

APPROACH:

1. Resident will h ave tasks assigned for each day of the week.
2. Resident will help out with one activity a day.
3. Resident will visit one other resident every day.
4. Resident will have an ongoing craft project.
5. Family will be asked to provide a VCR for the resident.

PROBLEM/NEED: (Misses animals)

1. Resident misses being responsible for pets and livestock.

GOAL:

1. Resident will feed nursing home pets daily.
2. Resident will help with monthly Humane Society pet visits.

APPROACH:

1. Resident will have pet food available to him and will keep the feeding schedules.
2. Resident will meet Humane Society pets and have them with him during visit and help in exhibiting them.

Example

Ms. M, an independent person, is having difficulty feeding herself because of tremors due to Parkinson's disease.

PROBLEM/NEED: (Wants independence)

1. Resident unhappy about the difficulty she has in feeding herself.

GOAL:

1. Resident will have special foods and equipment provided by (date) to make independent feeding possible.

APPROACH:

1. Rehabilitation specialists will evaluate resident by (date).
2. Food service will provide specially prepared food.
3. Social worker will work with resident to determine areas of concern.

BEHAVIOR

Example

Mr. N, a worrier, is prone to anxiety. As he finds himself in less control of circumstances and events his anxiety increases.

PROBLEM/NEED: (Anxiety)

1. Resident hyperventilates when he does not get his way.
2. Resident fears a heart attack because of palpitations and increased heart rate when he becomes anxious.
3. Resident worries he might do something wrong.
4. Resident worries that someone might disapprove of him.
5. Resident worries that family members have come to harm whenever they are not in his presence.
6. Resident becomes agitated and paces at meal times, fearing he will be late.
7. Resident requests constant reassurance.

GOAL:

1. Resident will learn to control hyperventilation three out of five times.
2. Resident will learn that heart symptoms are anxiety symptoms by (date).
3. Resident will learn one method to control anxiety by (date).
4. Resident will identify one thing he does right each day.
5. Resident will identify five people who like and approve of him.
6. Resident will call one family member one time a day for reassurance.
7. Resident will go to dining room whenever it is comfortable for him.
8. Resident will learn one way to reassure self by (date).
9. Resident will have evaluation by MD for medication to relieve anxiety by (date).

APPROACH:

1. Resident will be taught deep breathing techniques to short circuit physical symptoms caused by anxiety.
2. Resident will develop activities to distract him from his anxiety such as (reading, television, craft work, pet care, talking with a friend, exercise, writing).
3. (Nurse, social worker, doctor) will explain the symptoms of anxiety to the resident.
4. All staff will reassure resident that symptoms are from anxiety and not related to any physical problem at the time of each anxiety symptom.
5. Family and friends will be trained to reassure resident in a calm and convincing way.
6. Resident will have a special place in the dining room he can go to whenever he wants.
7. Resident will be taught relaxation techniques in weekly sessions.
8. Each day a designated staff member will meet with resident to determine what has gone right that day.
9. Resident will be helped to develop a list of people he trusts and whom he knows like him. He will continue to add to the list.
10. Family will help resident work out a weekly telephone schedule for contacting them.
11. An appointment will be made with MD for medication evaluation by (date).
12. Resident will have successes in controlling anxiety pointed out to him and be helped to use this knowledge of his own ability to control his anxiety. He will be taught how to reassure himself.
13. Activities, nurse, social worker will help resident learn to affirm his abilities and accomplishments and make positive statements about himself such as, "I can do it." "People like me." "I'm safe." "My family is fine."

Example

Ms. O suffers from Alzheimer's disease and is often disoriented. Because she misinterprets social cues she is prone to rapid and wide mood swings.

PROBLEM/NEED: **(Disoriented)**

1. Resident loses her glasses several times a day.
2. Resident looks for people who are no longer part of her life (mother, son, husband).
3. Resident constantly asks, "What time is it?"
4. Resident gets lost.

GOAL:

1. Resident will have a cord to keep glasses around her neck by (date).
2. Resident will reminisce about long gone family one time a day, instead of searching for them.
3. Resident will have a large clock in her room by (date).
4. Resident will find own room two times each day.

APPROACH:

1. Neck cord for glasses will be provided for resident by family by (date).
2. Staff members will ask about persons resident is seeking and engage resident in reminiscence about them each time she mentions them by asking questions, commenting on her feelings, or bringing up known facts.
3. Social worker will request that family provide clock for resident's room by (date).
4. Mealtimes and other important times will be prominently posted by resident's clock.
5. Resident's room will not be changed.
6. Resident's room door will have resident's name and a distinctive ornament.

7. Resident will be helped to find room before frustration develops.
8. Reality orientation approach will be used.

PROBLEM/NEED: **(Mood swings)**

1. Resident picks up mood of anyone around her.
2. Resident starts to cry for no apparent reason.
3. Resident is frequently verbally abusive during the evening shift.

GOAL:

1. Resident will be around cheerful, pleasant people whenever she is in a situation that can be controlled.
2. Resident will remain calm five out of seven evenings.

APPROACH:

1. Staff will always approach resident in a cheerful, pleasant, and positive manner.
2. Family will be helped to be upbeat and approving around resident.
3. Resident will attend remotivation group two times a week.
4. Resident will be helped out of uncomfortable situations by using redirection.
5. The validation approach will be used whenever resident is expressing distress.
6. Resident will be listened to when she expresses concern and her concerns will be validated.
7. Staff, family will give non-verbal recognition through pats, hugs, eye contact, smiles, nods.
8. Resident will get rest during every day so she is not too exhausted at night.
9. Resident will have night light to enhance visual cues when it is dark.

Example

Mr. P is an angry man who is sometimes verbally abusive and can get combative and physically aggressive. He is untrusting and suspicious of other people's motives and actions.

PROBLEM/NEED: (Angry, suspicious, abusive)

1. Resident never smiles.
2. Resident strikes out when touched.
3. Resident swears at other residents.
4. Resident criticizes nursing assistants' work.
5. Resident accuses bookkeeper of stealing from him.
6. Resident explosive and insulting to family members.
7. Resident throws his food on the floor.

GOAL:

1. Resident will smile one time per day.
2. Resident will not hit during morning activities of daily living care by (date).
3. Resident will not stay with other residents once swearing begins.
4. Resident will say, "Thank you," to nursing assistants one time a week.
5. Resident will receive monthly accounting of his funds.
6. Resident will be glad to see family fifteen minutes each week.
7. Resident will not throw food on floor for one meal per day.
8. Resident will learn one alternative method for handling anger.

APPROACH:

1. Staff and family will institute a behavior modification program. Resident will be rewarded for acceptable behavior and removed from hostile situations.
2. All procedures will be explained to resident before they are begun.

3. Resident will be evaluated by doctor for medication to ease agitation by (date).
4. Resident will be encouraged to discuss what makes him angry rather than to act out.
5. Resident will be taught to hit a pillow when upset.
6. Bookkeeper will prepare accounting of resident's finances for him each month.
7. Resident will be removed from area and returned to his room when he swears at other residents.
8. Resident will be asked to smile and/or say thank you when something is done to his liking. He will be given attention, praise, and recognition for doing so.
9. Family will be asked to not argue or be confrontive with resident, but to try to listen and agree and then leave when he gets verbally abusive.
10. Resident will be removed from dining room when food is thrown.
11. Staff members will listen to resident as long as he discusses feelings, but will leave when he becomes accusing.
12. Staff will anticipate resident's needs.
13. Resident will always be asked to agree to care.
14. Staff will not invade resident's personal boundaries except to give necessary care.
15. Staff will determine total pattern of agitation and note time, subject, person, activity, to be aware of what spawns problems for resident.
16. Social worker will help resident understand more constructive ways of obtaining what he wants by using the supportive approach.

Example

Ms. Q had always had someone to lean on and apparently plans to continue her dependent state. She manipulates staff, residents, and her family to get them to do things for her that she does not want to do for herself.

PROBLEM/NEED: **(Dependent)**

1. Resident wants nursing assistants to bathe and dress her although she can do this for herself.
2. Resident gets nursing home visitors to push her where she wants to go rather than exert herself.
3. Resident likes to get family members to make decisions for her.

GOAL:

1. Resident will wash her own face daily.
2. Resident will put on own outer garments.
3. Resident will get to dining room one time daily without help.
4. Resident will make one independent decision per week.

APPROACH:

1. Staff and family will praise and give attention to resident's independent actions.
2. Restorative techniques will be used to get resident to do one small independent action and progress small step by small step to more independent responsibilities.

   Examples:

   a. Resident will wash face after nursing assistant prepares wash cloth.
   b. Resident will prepare wash cloth and wash face.
   c. Resident will complete all preparations for washing face and wash her face.

   or

   a. Resident will have clothes laid out to put on.
   b. Resident will choose between two outfits and put one on.
   c. Resident will make own selection and put on outer garments.

   or

    a. Resident will be given two alternatives and asked to select one.

    b. Resident will be given all alternatives and expected to make a decision.

    c. Resident will discuss choices, explore alternatives, and make a decision.

or

    a. Staff member will walk with resident while she pushes herself to dining room

    b. Staff member will advise resident that it is time to wheel self to dining room and supervise from a distance.

    c. Resident will take self to dining room.

3. Family will be helped to work as a team member in encouraging resident's independence and decision making. Their efforts will be positively reinforced.

PROBLEM/NEED; (Manipulative)

1. Resident hints at what she wants, rather than ask directly.
2. Resident exaggerates needs in order to get attention and assistance.
3. Resident acts helpless and makes family feel that they should do more for her.

GOAL:

1. Resident will ask for what she wants directly one time a day.
2. Resident will learn to get attention by independent activity by (date).
3. Resident will tell family of one accomplishment by (date).

APPROACH:

1. Staff will not respond to hints.
2. Staff will help resident restate her hint into a direct request. Staff will respond to the direct request.

3. Resident will be given positive reinforcement for action and accomplishment.
4. Family will be helped to handle their guilt and take a more constructive approach with resident.
5. Resident will have progress pointed out to her. She will be helped to tell her family of her progress.

Example

Mr. R resists anything uncomfortable to him, but is particularly upset by bath time. He not only yells, but sometimes he fights and ends up with scratches and bruises.

PROBLEM/NEED: (Fear of bath)

1. Resident becomes upset when faced with a bath, sometimes hurting himself in his agitation.

GOAL:

1. Resident will have sponge baths five days a week.
2. Resident will accept one bath per week.

APPROACH:

1. Resident will be given sponge baths in his room.
2. Resident will have explanations of procedure each step of the way.
3. Resident will be bathed at optimum time of the day - his choice.
4. Resident will be approached pleasantly, calmly, and reassuringly.
5. Staff will use a positive approach to help resident see the bath as a pleasant experience.
6. Resident's family will be told of bath problem so that they can understand what has been happening with resident and support staff in their efforts.

Example

Ms. S is bedridden and unresponsive.

PROBLEM/NEED: (Unresponsive)

1. Resident is no longer receiving frequent family visits.

2. Resident does not give feed-back.

GOAL:

1. Resident will have family visits one time a week.
2. Resident will respond with one non-verbal signal when pleasantly stimulated.

APPROACH:

1. Family will be helped to understand what is going on with the resident and how to spend visiting times giving comfort and good feelings through music, pleasant speech, and touch.
2. Staff will work with resident daily to get resident to respond to touch with hand or eye movement or sounds of contentment.

Example

Mr. T, a strong believer in home remedies, not only likes to treat himself, but refuses to see a physician.

PROBLEM/NEED: (Refuses to see doctor)

1. Resident has a cold and refuses a medical evaluation.

GOAL:

1. Resident will see doctor by (date).

APPROACH:

1. Medical regulations will be explained to resident.
2. Residents who have seen the physician will talk to resident.
3. Social worker will talk with resident to determine if there are any fears that need to be explored.
4. Resident will get to meet the doctor on a casual basis.

Example

Ms. U is extremely thin. She needs to gain weight, not only to look better, but for her physical well being.

PROBLEM/NEED: (Malnourished)

1. Resident does not demonstrate an interest in food.
2. Resident only likes sweets.

3. Resident eats treats brought by family and refuses regular meals.
4. Unless supervised, resident just plays with her food.

GOAL:
1. Resident will eat seventy-five percent of all meals.
2. Resident will have nutritious treats daily.
3. Resident will eat sweets only after meals or on special occasions.
4. Resident will eat with supervision.

APPROACH:
1. Resident's food likes and dislikes will be explored.
2. Resident will be fed at regular two hour intervals to help her develop an eating habit.
3. Family will be counseled on types of foods to bring resident to assist her in achieving optimum health.
4. Resident will have company during each meal to encourage her to eat and enjoy her food.
5. Resident will be served sweets only after other nutritional requirements have been met.

Example

Mr. V has a short attention span. He cannot keep his mind on one subject or focus on one thing at a time if there is more than one stimulus to capture his attention.

PROBLEM/NEED: (Distractible)
1. Resident cannot follow program of any group activity as he cannot focus on the major event.
2. Resident forgets what he sets out to do.
3. Resident asks the same question over and over, forgetting the answer.

GOAL:
1. Resident will have one individual activity per day.

2. Resident will receive assistance in completing necessary tasks of daily living.
3. Resident will have all his questions answered with patience and understanding.

APPROACH:

1. (Volunteer, family, staff member) will participate with resident in one mutual activity a day. Through this activity he will have the pleasure of companionship, achievement, and self-esteem.
2. Resident will have assistance to follow through on any necessary task.
3. All resident's questions will be answered completely and with courtesy.

Example

Ms. W suffers from a delusion that someone is going to come into her room at night and hurt her.

PROBLEM/NEED: (Delusion)

1. Resident is afraid to go to bed at night because of her fear of an intruder.
2. When resident sees curtains flutter she is sure someone is breaking in.

GOAL:

1. Resident will be placed in a room without windows by (date).
2. Curtains will be removed from the resident's window by (date) and replaced with more stable window coverings.
3. Resident will feel secure in room by (date).

APPROACH:

1. Resident will be moved to an inside room.
2. Blinds will be installed in place of curtains in resident's room.
3. Cross-bars will be installed on resident's window.
4. Social worker will help resident discuss fears and assure her she will be safe and protected.

5. Resident will be evaluated by physician for night medication.

Example

Mr. X has difficulty making friends because he whines and complains about his health.

PROBLEM/NEED: **(Complains about physical health)**

1. Resident concentrates the majority of his attention on his physical symptoms.
2. Resident frequently refuses activities because of physical complaints.
3. Other residents get tired of hearing about resident's health and avoid him.

GOAL:

1. Resident will confine complaints regarding his physical health to the morning and evening hours.
2. Resident will attend one activity at least one-half way through per day.
3. Resident will have one topic of conversation, other than his health, each day.

APPROACH:

1. Staff will listen to resident's complaints in the morning and the evening, but redirect any mention of health problems in the afternoon.
2. Resident will have all health concerns met in the morning and evening. Other topics will be proposed in the afternoon.
3. Resident will be taken to activities and helped to stay at least half way through, and assisted to leave when he gets uncomfortable.
4. Social worker will work with resident to help him understand other topics of conversation are needed to make friends.

Example

Mr. Y wanders away from the facility.

PROBLEM/NEED: **(Wanders)**

1. Resident goes out the front door and gets lost and disoriented.

2. Resident tries to run away from the facility.

GOAL:

1. Resident will not leave the facility without supervision.

APPROACH:

1. Resident will be kept busy in the facility with activities, meals, and projects.
2. (Staff, family, volunteers) will take resident for daily supervised walks.
3. If tolerated a bell will be put on resident's wheelchair so his whereabouts can be readily determined.

Example

Ms. Z has episodes of unreality. Occasionally she is observed talking with someone who is not present.

PROBLEM/NEED: (Hallucinations)

1. Resident frightens other residents when she holds conversations with people they cannot see.
2. Resident confuses reality and unreality, sometimes accusing staff members of saying or doing something they did not say or do.

GOAL:

1. Resident will be evaluated by a psychiatrist by (date).
2. Resident will not be around other residents when she is hallucinating.
3. Resident will not accuse staff during morning shift.

APPROACH:

1. Staff will not argue or get defensive with resident.
2. Staff will always observe the resident's personal boundaries.
3. Staff will be reassuring and understanding with resident, but also truthful and realistic.
4. Psychiatric evaluation will be arranged by (date).

MATERIAL NEEDS

Example

Mr. AA is not satisfied with nursing home fare and wants the snacks he is accustomed to.

PROBLEM/NEED: (Special treats)

1. Resident wants mints after meals.
2. Resident likes fresh fruit for afternoon snacks.
3. Resident insists on pizza one time a week.
4. Resident wants "home-made" cookies.
5. Resident enjoys chewing gum.

GOAL:

1. Resident will have the snack of his choice three times a day.

APPROACH:

1. Snacks will be kept for resident at (place).
2. Family will be asked to supply resident's needs.
3. (Staff member) will monitor stock of snacks.

Example

Ms. BB is no longer safe in a wheelchair and needs a specially designed geri-chair for comfort and security.

PROBLEM/NEED: (Special Aids)

1. Resident runs into walls and people with wheelchair.
2. Resident slides down in wheelchair.

GOAL:

1. Resident will have a geri-chair by (date).

APPROACH:

1. Relatives will be asked to provide needed geri-chair.
2. Physician will provide prescription for chair.

Example

Mr. CC has a nephew handling his affairs. There is some question that the nephew might be exploiting the resident's finances. Mr. CC has expressed concern.

PROBLEM/NEED: (Exploitation)

1. Resident is worried about his funds being mishandled.
2. Resident complains about nephew to staff, but fears confrontation with him.

GOAL:

1. Resident will switch financial management from nephew to (attorney, bank, financial manager, another relative) by (date).
2. Resident will confer with the State Adult Protection Agency regarding fears of exploitation by (date).
3. Resident will discuss exploitation with the State's Attorney by (date).
4. Resident will obtain a guardian by (date).

APPROACH:

1. Resident will discuss problem with nursing home social worker.
2. Social worker will present alternatives to resident, i.e., state protective service investigation, state's attorney filing charges, transferring management to an attorney, bank, qualified, individual, or having a guardian appointed.
3. Social worker will make arrangements for resident to follow course of his choice.

Example

Mr. DD broke his hip, came to the nursing home for care and therapy, is doing well, and plans to be in the nursing home for a short period of time.

PROBLEM/NEED: (Short term placement)

1. Resident is planning to leave at the end of three months.
2. Resident does not want to get involved with nursing home routine and activities.

GOAL:

1. Resident will have ongoing needs met at time of discharge.
2. Resident will have one interesting thing to do each day.

APPROACH:

1. Social worker will make discharge plans and arrange for follow-up home delivered services.
2. Family will be prepared to meet resident's needs at time of discharge.
3. Resident's likes and dislikes will be determined and he will be scheduled for group and individual activities one time a day to fill his time and occupy his interest.

Example

Mr. EE is worried. His funds are depleted and he wonders how to pay for his care.

PROBLEM/NEED: (Finances depleted)

1. Resident can no longer pay his own nursing home bill.

GOAL:

1. Resident will be approved for Medicaid payment for nursing home care by (date).

APPROACH:

1. Social worker will help family apply for Medicaid funds from the state to pay for resident's care.

Example

Ms. FF likes to attend church, a club meeting, and the epilepsy group meetings outside the facility. Nursing home transportation is not always available.

PROBLEM/NEED: (Transportation)

1. Resident gets upset if she does not get out of facility for church.
2. Resident gets cranky if she does not get to her club meeting.
3. Resident feels deprived if epilepsy group transportation is not provided for her.

GOAL:

1. Resident will have transportation to two events per week.

APPROACH:

1. Social worker will talk with relatives about providing transportation.
2. Council on Aging will be asked to provide transportation.
3. Volunteer services will be explored to determine availability of transportation.

RELATIONSHIPS

Example

Ms. GG misses her family. They live out of state and can visit only one time a year.

PROBLEM/NEED: (Infrequent family visits)

1. Resident expresses frequent desire to be more involved with her family.

GOAL:

1. Resident will telephone family monthly.
2. Resident will write family weekly.

APPROACH:

1. Social worker will telephone family by (date) to arrange monthly telephone calls.
2. Family will be sent the facility monthly newsletter.
3. Family will be asked to write bi-weekly.
4. Resident will be helped to write weekly.
5. Facility staff will send out quarterly up-dates to family.
6. Family will be encouraged to send pictures and videos to resident.

Example

Ms. HH has roommate problems. She does not like her roommate. They do not get along. They fight over space, room use, privacy.

PROBLEM/NEED: (Does not get along with roommate)

1. Resident accuses roommate of putting things on her side of the room.
2. Resident complains that roommate has too many visitors.
3. Resident unhappy that she never gets time alone in her room.

GOAL:

1. Resident will be relocated with compatible roommate by (date).

2. All resident's clothes, closets, and drawers will be labeled and space delineated by (date).
3. Resident and roommate will have other specified areas in the nursing home for visiting and entertaining.
4. Resident's needs for privacy will be noted and privacy times arranged by (date).

APPROACH:

1. A new roommate will be selected for resident's consideration by (date).
2. Resident's and roommate's belongings will be sorted out, labeled, put in storage, and space evenly divided by (date).
3. Resident's and roommate's visitors will understand that they will use an assigned area outside the room for visiting times.
4. Resident's and roommate's use of room will be monitored to determine if each has time to be alone. Depending on the outcome other adjustments and arrangements may be made.

Example

Mr. II's roommate died. He is missing him and is not accepting a new roommate.

PROBLEM/NEED: (Roommate dies)

1. Resident misses roommate who died.
2. Resident has stopped attending activities he used to attend with his roommate.
3. Resident wants to talk about his roommate.

GOAL:

1. Resident will meet one other compatible person by (date).
2. Resident will attend one new activity each week.
3. Resident will have someone to talk with about his roommate three times a week.

APPROACH:

1. Resident will be introduced to other residents with similar abilities and interests.
2. Resident will be invited to attend other activities so he can keep busy until he is ready to go to old favored activities.
3. (Volunteer, family, staff member, other residents) will be available to listen and to reminisce about resident's roommate and friend.

PROBLEM/NEED: (Will not accept roommate)

1. Resident tells roommate he does not belong in room.
2. Resident insults roommate.
3. Whenever roommate enters the room, resident leaves.

GOAL:

1. Resident will help select a roommate he can accept by (date).
2. Resident will learn and acknowledge two things he likes about the present roommate by (date).
3. Resident and roommate will find one activity to attend together by (date).

APPROACH:

1. Possible roommates will be proposed to resident.
2. Social worker will help resident find some things he likes about his roommate.
3. Mutual interests will be explored and activities the roommates can do together will be arranged.

Example

Ms. JJ expects her roommate to do as she demands. This includes times to go to bed and get up, running errands for Ms. JJ, when she must turn off the television, and even who she should have as friends.

PROBLEM/NEED: (Orders roommate around)

1. Resident expects roommate to take care of her.

2. Resident dominates roommate.

GOAL:

1. Resident will accept daily care from staff.
2. Resident will be involved in two activities separate from her roommate each day.

APPROACH:

1. It will be made clear to resident that she and her roommate are both to receive care from nursing home staff.
2. Roommate will be stopped from running errands for resident whenever it is noted that she is doing so. Resident or staff will perform the task instead.
3. Roommate will be introduced to other people and assisted to attend mutually satisfying events with them.
4. Resident will be taken from her room to two events each day.
5. A television schedule will be worked out and posted. It will be one that is a fair compromise between the resident and her roommate.

Example

Mr. KK sees the Resident's Council as his private forum. He dominates it with complaints. Other residents share some of his concerns, but are irritated, intimidated, and outraged at his demeanor.

PROBLEM/NEED: (Dominates Residents' Council)

1. Resident drives others away from attending Residents' Council meeting by his overpowering behavior.
2. Resident does not give others a chance to speak in Residents' Council.
3. No one knows how to handle resident during Residents' Council meeting. He takes over the meeting.

GOAL:

1. Resident will have fifteen minutes to air complaints during Residents' Council meetings.

2. Resident will be kept busy during Residents' Council meetings, taking the minutes.
3. Resident will air complaints in between meetings to appropriate personnel.

APPROACH:

1. Social worker will discuss residents complaints with him two times a week.
2. Resident's complaints will have a response so he will see the effectiveness of complaining appropriately.
3. Resident will be asked to take minutes at the Residents' Council meetings.
4. Social worker will help resident write up documented complaints to be presented in an orderly manner.

Example

Ms. LL is fifty-seven years old, but because of physical problems, needs nursing home care. Because she is so much younger than the rest of the residents she does not have much in common with them.

PROBLEM/NEED: (Younger resident)

1. Resident does not want to attend activities geared to older residents.
2. Resident gets moody about living with so many older people.

GOAL:

1. Resident will do volunteer work inside the nursing home one time a week.
2. Resident will do volunteer work outside nursing home one time a week.
3. Resident will join an organization or club by (date).

APPROACH:

1. Resident will volunteer to help staff, to help in activities, or to help with special projects and will have rewarding responsibilities.

2. Resident will work as a tutor, work with the learn to read program as an instructor, or in some other volunteer activity where she will meet people and be needed.
3. Resident will be involved in a group or organization of her choice. Transportation to the meetings will be arranged for her.
4. Social worker will meet bi-weekly with resident to help her make satisfactory use of her time.

Example

Mr. MM was an only child. He and his wife had no children. They moved to this locality from another state. Mr. MM became a widower and then a nursing home resident. He has no visitors and no one to take care of his special desires.

PROBLEM/NEED: (No relatives or friends)

1. Resident has no visitors.
2. Resident wants jelly beans on hand at all times.

GOAL:

1. Resident will have one visitor per week.
2. Resident will have his jelly beans available to him at all times.

APPROACH:

1. Resident will have a volunteer visit weekly.
2. Minister and church members will be asked to visit.
3. A foster grandchild will be assigned.
4. (Volunteer, staff member) will shop and have jelly beans in the nursing home and available for resident.

Example

Ms. NN's family apparently cares for her. They visit regularly. They agree to do whatever she asks of them. But they hate to upset her so they sneak away instead of saying good-bye. They do not always keep their promises or do what they say they will do for her. They appease her, but do not follow through.

PROBLEM/NEED: (Family does not keep promises)

1. Resident is still waiting for the family outing she was promised.

2. Resident does not dare let family out of sight as they sneak off when she is not looking.

GOAL:

1. Resident will have family outing by (date) or family will tell her that there will not be a family outing.
2. Resident's family will always say good-bye to resident before they leave the facility.

APPROACH:

1. Social worker will plan resident's outing with family.
2. Social worker will explain how important it is for resident to know what is to be done and that false promises just build up unfulfilled expectations.
3. Social worker will help family say good-bye to resident after every visit.
4. Social worker will meet with family to help them work through their own feelings.

Example

Mr. OO is in love. He has a girl-friend who also lives in the facility. His problem is that they never seem to be able to be alone to get better acquainted, to talk, to be affectionate.

PROBLEM/NEED: (Need for privacy)

1. Resident distressed as he feels there is nowhere he and his girl-friend can go and not be interrupted.

GOAL:

1. Resident and his girl-friend will have one hour of privacy one day per week.

APPROACH:

1. A private place, i.e., resident's room, conference room, activity room, will be reserved for resident and girl-friend for one hour at a set time each week.

SOME COMMENTS ON CARE PLANS

Obviously these care plans are not all inclusive. They are meant to give you an idea of the varied problems, goals, and approaches a social worker might select to help a resident with his or her unique concern.

The key is unique. Each individual is just that — an individual. The same approach may work differently with each person. Unlike a medical or dietary problem, there is no one prescribed way to handle a social or emotional problem. Much depends on the resident's personality and ability.

SECTION III
HELP FOR THE HELPER

QUARTERLY PROGRESS NOTES

Quarterly progress notes are not only required, but give a picture of the resident's current status. Are there changes? Have the residents progressed or regressed? To make progress notes meaningful and useful for planning, consider the following areas.

1. Review concerns of the other disciplines.
2. Note the residents' deficits (vision, hearing, speech, ambulation) and how to help them compensate for these losses.
3. What are the relationships with: - staff/volunteers?
   - other residents?
   - family/friends?
4. Follow up on the care plans. Were they carried out? How successful have the approaches been?
5. Is the discharge plan correct and backed up with data?
6. Are there special concerns or needs?
7. Include strengths to work with or build on.
8. How does the past (before nursing home) effect present behavior (i.e., work, marriage, sickness, children)?

When writing the progress note up-dates include:

PHYSICAL
   Handicaps and how residents handle them
   Ambulation status
   Activities of daily living
   Degree of comfort/discomfort
   Aids, i.e., glasses, hearing aids

SOCIAL
   Friends
   Family
   Relationships with staff, other residents, roommate
   Finances

Material needs
Support system

BEHAVIORAL
Communication
Eating/sleeping
Activities
Preferences
Withdrawn/acting out

EMOTIONAL
Moods
Aggressive/passive
Happy/sad
Adjustment
Spiritual

CARE PLAN
Problem and goal
What doing in regard to problem
Results

DISCHARGE
Discharge status and why

QUARTERLY PROGRESS NOTE FORM

An alternative to written, summarized quarterly progress notes is a summary form. Progress note entries can still be made for incidents and events that occur between quarterly up-dates or for complicated and/or traumatic situations that require more detailed explanation.

A quarterly summary form is included. It is an example of a form that is acceptable and effective. The summary is particularly useful for charting and noting changes in the residents. To make it meaningful it is essential to elaborate in the remarks column. Just using the check list does not give the full picture or indicate your full knowledge of the residents' functioning.

SOCIAL SERVICE QUARTERLY SUMMARY

DATE_____ RESIDENT'S NAME_____

PHYSICAL
HEARING   REMARKS
___Good___With___Without hearing aid   _____
___Impaired___With___Without hearing aid   _____
VISION
___Good___With___Without glasses   _____
___Impaired___With___Without glasses   _____
___Makes eye contact   _____
AMBULATION
___Good___With___Without aids   _____
___Impaired___With Without aids   _____
PAIN
___None___Controlled___Chronic___Severe   _____
GROOMING
___Good___Poor___Resists   _____
___Grooms self___Needs help with _____   _____
SPEECH
___Good___Impaired because of_____   _____
___Communicates by_____   _____
___Makes needs known___Rambles___Talks constantly   _____
HEALTH PROBLEMS
___Terminal illness___Progressive disease   _____
___Needs monitoring___Fragile health   _____
___Uncooperative with medical management   _____

BEHAVIORAL
BEHAVIOR
___Abusive___Agreeable___Aggressive___Agitated   _____
___Belligerent___Complaining___Cooperative   _____
___Crying___Demanding___Excitable___Friendly   _____
___Gregarious___Moody___Outgoing___Participates   _____
___Passive___Private___Responsible___Smiling   _____
___Sociable___Touchy___Unreasonable___Withdrawn   _____
___Yells   _____
ORIENTATION
___Person___Place___Time   _____

EMOTIONAL
MOOD
___Anxious___Bored___Cheerful___Confused___Content   _____
___Crabby___Depressed___Fearful___Happy___Irritable   _____
___Jealous___Joyful___Labile___Nervous___Pleasant   _____
___Sad___Worried   _____
MEDICATION
___For anxiety___For depression___For psychosis   _____
___For agitation   _____

Room No._____ Patient Record No._____ Physician_____

Hughes and Espinosa

ADJUSTMENT	REMARKS
___Tries to leave NH___Dislikes NH	
___Accepts NH___Considers NH home	

SOCIAL
FRIENDS
___None___Visit sporadically___Visit regularly
___Call___Write
FAMILY
___Parent___Spouse___Children___Other___None
___Visit sporadically___Visit regularly___Call
___Write___Supportive___Critical___Need help
OTHER RESIDENTS
___Affable___No relationships___Few special friends
___Aggravates others___Refuses to socialize
ROOMMATE
___Good relationship___Some Problems
___Antagonistic relationship___No relationship
ACTIVITIES
___Solitary___One to one___Groups___Spectator
___Hand work___Exercise___Learning___Music
___Parties___Reminiscence___Talking___Information
FINANCES
___Adequate___Needs help___Problems
STAFF
___Good relationship___Tolerates staff
___Antagonistic
RELIGION
___Active with_____
___Clergy visits___Church members visit___Inactive

CARE PLAN
Problems resolved_____
Ongoing problems_____
New Problems_____
Goals_____
Approaches_____

DISCHARGE
___Planning for discharge___Referrals
___Other placement___Contingent on health
___Planning longer term care

OTHER _____
_____
_____
_____

COMMENTS _____
_____
_____
_____
_____

SOCIAL WORKER'S SIGNATURE_____

PSYCHOSOCIAL APPROACHES

All approaches do not work for everyone. Several approaches can be used at the same time. The following specialized approaches have been effective in restoring dignity and helping the residents be happier and more acceptable in their behavior.

Reality Orientation

(Orient the residents to time, place and person.)

Reality Orientation is a technique to be used daily by everyone who spends time with the residents. The specific set of ideas to be followed are:

1. Provide a calm environment.
2. Maintain a set routine.
3. Give clear, simple responses to the resident's questions and clear, simple questions when asking something of the residents.
4. Talk clearly, not loudly, to residents.
5. Give directions clearly and succinctly. Do not give explanations as they distract from the message. If need be, guide the resident to and from the destination.
6. Remind them of the date, time, place, and person.
7. Do not let them stay confused by allowing them to ramble in their speech and actions.
8. Be firm, but kind and courteous.
9. Be sincere.
10. Be consistent.
11. Treat with dignity and respect.
12. Treat resident like the adult they are.
13. Talk with residents as though you expect them to understand. Explain details slowly. Give time to comprehend. Take time to listen and understand.
14. Do not hurry the residents.

15. Take time to explain each new procedure before asking the residents to do it.
16. It helps to act out, to demonstrate, what is to be done.
17. Allow residents to do all they can for themselves. Assist and encourage only when necessary.

Validation

(Be with the residents in time, place, and feeling)

This approach was formulated and pioneered by Naomi Feil. For more thorough information see her book "Validation: The Feil Method" (Edward Feil Productions, 1982).

In validation the residents' feelings are accepted. The person with the residents acknowledges the feelings, sometimes mirrors them, and encourages free expression. The feelings are not discouraged, criticized, forced, or analyzed. Even though the residents are experiencing feelings about a long past event they are seen as true, meaningful, and current.

The staff member:

1. Lets the residents know she hears and accepts what the residents are saying and feeling.
2. Helps the residents express their feelings.
3. Is comforting and accepting, using voice and manner to convey this.
4. Understands that the residents are working through feelings about past events that need resolution.
5. Concentrates on the feelings, realizing that the facts are unimportant.
6. Uses intuition and compassion to put feelings into words.
7. Never criticizes or corrects.
8. Sometimes acts out the feelings with the residents, using their actions, such as pacing or pounding.

9. Recognizes that the feelings are significant to the residents and does nothing to make them insignificant.
10. Uses touch to make contact and convey assurance.

Self-Esteem Enhancement

(Praise and recognition of the residents' worth)

Self-esteem makes it possible for the residents to have dignity, enjoy life, and tolerate others because the residents feel good about themselves. Methods for enhancing self-esteem are discussed in the book "Enhancing the Self Esteem of the Nursing Home Resident" by Marylou Hughes (M & H Publishing Company, 1987).

Self-esteem is enhanced by concentrating on the residents' positive assets, helping them feel worthwhile, and creating a sense of independence.

Approaches to enhance self-esteem are to:

1. Recognize and accept the residents' values. Even though we may not agree with the residents' priorities, we accept them as theirs and of value.
2. Let the residents know we are happy to be around them..
3. Ask for and accept their opinions.
4. Give encouragement, approval, recognition.
5. Acknowledge their presence, their contributions.
6. Give special notice.
7. Pay attention to their environment. Keep it neat, clean, and cheerful.
8. Provide treats.
9. Arrange pleasant and interesting events and relationships.
10. Compliment sincerely.
11. Help them be as independent as they can be.
12. Help them look as good as they can.

Restorative Techniques

(Assist residents to do what they can do)

The restorative approach recognizes that any ability the residents have can be used to further their physical and mental health and lead them towards a more fulfilled life. An example of the restorative approach is resocialization as discussed in this book beginning on page 117. With restoration we start with what the residents can do and enlarge their life and environment by adding to it or using the skill in another way that gives new experiences and a positive attitude.

The restorative approach goes as follows:

1. The residents can sit up, but cannot walk. They use a wheelchair.
2. Since they can sit they are helped to sit in other areas out of their wheelchairs.
3. The residents are seated on chairs in the dining room instead of being wheeled up to the table.
4. This gives the residents a feeling of independence because they sit at the table as they did in earlier years and as other people do. They become more sociable and more willing to try other things.
5. By changing one pattern in behavior and/or ability, other areas in the residents' lives are enhanced. For example, sitting on a regular chair in a dining room encourages appetite, friendships, independence, and leads to more interest in grooming.

Non-Verbal Communication

(Signal approval, caring, and happiness)

Non-verbal communication is our most powerful and effective means of letting people know what we feel and think. We retain stronger memories of how people act towards us than we do of what they say to us.

To give positive non-verbal communication:

1. Make eye contact.
2. Look at people while you listen.
3. Touch gently and with affection.
4. Smile.
5. Nod with approval.
6. Indicate recognition.
7. Look happy to see them.
8. Look attentive.
9. Move closer.

Distraction

(Change direction to more constructive feelings or behavior)

When residents are focused on something that is making them unhappy or are in a miserable mood, by changing the subject, your attitude, or the environment, you can distract the residents and change their outlook.

To use distraction do not negate the residents' feelings, but do help them control their feelings by:

1. Moving them to a more cheerful area if someone or something is bothering them where they are.
2. Approaching them with a positive attitude and happy countenance to make them feel good about themselves and others.
3. Taking their attention from whatever is unsatisfactory to something they like or enjoy.
4. Getting them involved in something that requires concentration such as hand work, catching a ball, singing, sorting, turning the pages of a book.

Reassurance

(Accept, attempt to understand, and comfort)

Reassurance is a technique that is used to diminish fears by letting the residents know that good outcomes are usual and can be expected. Reassurance is written up in more detail in the book "Mental Health Problems and the Nursing Home Resident" on pages 26, 27, and 28, by Marylou Hughes (M & H Publishing Company, Inc., 1988).

To be reassuring, staff members:

1. Listen to the residents' concerns.
2. Accept the residents' concerns.
3. Try to understand the concerns through clarification and exploration of the problem.
4. Stay with the residents as long as they need reassurance.
5. Give them correct information and clear up misconceptions.
6. Give positive suggestions regarding their abilities and knowledge.
7. Assure residents that help is available.
8. Point out what has gone well and can be expected to go well again.
9. Act confident, helpful, and trustworthy.
10. Are available when needed.

Participation

(Involve residents in doing)

Participating and being part of events is a much more satisfactory state of being than to be an outside observer. The more residents participate, the more they develop a sense of belonging and a stake in what goes on in their environment. Being a part of something connotes inclusion and competence. To use participation, staff members can:

1. Give the residents choices.
2. Ask them to do as much as they can do for themselves.
3. Include them in planning.
4. Assign tasks to help in entertainment, publicity, or nursing home administration.

5. Work along with them.
6. Help them help others.
7. Involve them in problem solving.

Supportive

(Give non-threatening guidance)

Being supportive is to give emotional assistance through encouragement, guidance, suggestion, advice, explanation, and persuasion. The residents may badly need encouragement to conquer fears and do what they really want to do. They may need guidance in the form of understanding the alternatives in order to make a choice they can live with. Sometimes a desirable outcome must be suggested, or advice given that is based on knowledge. Explanations of what can happen or what is to be expected diminish anxiety. Persuasion to try or to do the right thing may be needed.

The supportive staff member is:

1. Available.
2. Comforting.
3. Encouraging to residents who need to take small risks in order to enrich their lives.
4. Understanding.
5. Reassuring.
6. Able to explain what is happening and why it is happening.
7. Able to answer questions in a clear manner that lets the residents feel they have a right to know.
8. Present when needed.

Re-direct

(Help residents out of untenable situations)

Residents may get confrontive or argumentative or take a stand and then not know how to back out of an uncomfortable and potentially dangerous situation. They are not able to shift gears quickly or are concerned about saving face. To re-direct is to help the residents regain their composure and keep their ego intact.

Staff members re-direct by:

1. Acknowledging the residents' positions.
2. Letting the residents know that their feelings are legitimate.
3. Giving the residents an alternative thought or action.
4. If need be, insisting that the residents are needed elsewhere.

Listening

(Give active attention and listen to the residents)

There is no more flattering action than to give undivided attention. Older residents sometimes take longer to formulate and express a thought. Staff members need to stay attentive and occasionally direct the residents' thoughts and ask questions to help them make their points and express their concerns. The assistance and the questions show that the staff member is listening and trying to understand. When someone listens it makes people feel more secure, cherished, important, and gives them a better feeling about themselves and their surroundings.

To be an active listener:

1. Ask questions. Do not jump to conclusions. Hear the residents out.
2. Keep an open mind.
3. Make note of the emotions that accompany the message.
4. Try to capture the residents' point of view.
5. Be attentive. Act as though being with them is the most important thing you have to do.
6. Use encouraging sounds such as uh huh, go on, and ask, then what.
7. Rephrase what the residents said to make sure you really heard what they said.

See pages 125 and 126 of "The Nursing Home and the Resident's Relatives" by Marylou Hughes (M & H Publishing Company, 1987) for more information on active listening.

Anticipation of Needs

(Set schedule and take care of wants and needs of residents)

Residents who cannot make their needs known will become agitated when their needs are not met. To deter upsets, they can be kept comfortable by making sure their needs are taken care of before the need is there. Anticipating needs means that essentials are attended to before concern arises and a schedule that can be counted on is adhered to.

Anticipating needs is effective when:

1. Normal needs are considered and carefully attended. These needs include clothing, room temperature, refreshments, comfort, entertainment, personal care and bathing, toileting, and grooming.
2. The residents' individual needs and preferences are realized and routinely given attention.
3. The schedule is predictable, comfortable, inevitable, and does not vary.
4. The needs to be anticipated are written down with method, place, and time of delivery known.

See page 126 and 127 of "The Nursing Home and the Resident's Relatives" by Marylou Hughes (M & H Publishing Company, 1987) for more on anticipating needs.

Behavior Modification

(Mold behavior through reinforcing desired responses)

Behavior modification is a technique which has the purpose of assisting individuals modify behavior that stands in the way of optimum functioning. The following explains the steps used in applying this technique.

1. Identify the behavior you want to change.
2. Analyze the behavior. When does it happen? Who is around when it happens? What is going on when it happens? HOW OFTEN DOES IT HAPPEN?!

3. Find out what is important to the person. What would be the reward that would be effective? Do not neglect the rewards of attention, praise, and touching.

4. Make the reward occur immediately after the behavior you want to reinforce occurs. If necessary set up a situation in which the desired behavior happens.

5. Make sure that all the staff know what is going on, and why, so everyone can be consistent.

6. Keep a record.

General Information on Behavior Modification

1. There is a danger that unwanted behavior may become much worse before it gets better. This happens because the usual behavior is not getting the usual response. Consequently, the person tries harder for a period of time. If there continues to be no response the behavior will disappear.

2. Keep in mind that any behavior that is rewarded will continue.

3. Rules are needed to define appropriate behavior.

4. Approval responses include verbal praise, physical contact, and body language.

5. Inappropriate behavior should be ignored, if at all possible.

6. When there is inappropriate behavior that cannot be ignored, use a negative response instead of punishment. Negative responses include verbal disapproval, and body language which indicates displeasure with the behavior. The offender may need removal from the situation.

7. Let every member of the team have a part. This includes outside professionals and family.

8. Negative responses may be necessary in instances of property damage, hurting others, acting out, or constantly irritating behavior.

9. There may need to be role playing so that the person knows what behavior is acceptable.

10. All rules, or expected behaviors, must be positive, stated concisely, be consistent, be precise, and must be rules that will be upheld. The fewer rules, the better.

11. Praise, or give a negative response to the behavior, not to the person. For example: The behavior is good or bad, the person is not condemned.

12. Use four positive responses to every one negative response. If negatives are used more than twenty-five percent of the time you are reinforcing negative behavior.

13. List the behaviors you can ignore, and those you cannot.

14. Help the residents find some other means of expressing feelings, rather than acting out, through role playing situations or allowing them to talk about their feelings or saying how you might feel under similar circumstances.

15. Behavior nearing what you want should be praised.

Modeling

(Demonstrate the wanted behavior)

When staff members show residents how to handle a situation the residents can gain confidence in their own ability while learning more constructive methods of interacting with others. Staff members can model cheerfulness, respect for others, confidence, and tact. This sets the tone for the residents.

Modeling behavior:

1. Exhibits a polite demeanor that respects individual rights and privacy.

2. Shows consideration for others' behaviors and viewpoints.

3. Is firm when need be as there are times when residents must be immediately shown a better way to approach a situation.

4. Is not critical of the residents' behavior, but demonstrates an improved approach.

Reminiscence

(Talk about, acknowledge, enjoy, and learn from the residents' report on the past)

Many approaches are incorporated into reminiscence. Listening, enhancing self-esteem, validation, non-verbal communication, and support are all a part of helping residents reminisce. Reminiscence gives the residents recognition for being whole persons with interesting pasts. It helps them enjoy their life and build on what they have done. It affirms them. It gives them pleasure as they recall accomplishments and memorable times.

To be part of the residents' reminiscence:

1. Show interest in their memories.
2. Try to learn about the residents' lives and about history through their life reviews.
3. Ask specific questions about past holidays, prices, ways of doing things.
4. Accept their memories as facts. Do not try to correct or challenge them.
5. Learn what their interests were and build on them by bringing those interests into the present.
6. Use what is learned about the residents through reminiscence to continue conversations on subjects that interest them.
7. Remember what was told and bring it up so that residents can relive favorite moments again and again.
8. Refrain from telling the residents that you have heard that story before.

INVOLVING FAMILIES AND THE COMMUNITY

It is good public relations and it is good for the resident and staff to have more people involved and interested. It helps everyone.

To include families and the community in the provision of resident care consider some of the following.

1. Invite family members to care plan meetings by approaching them personally and sending written invitations.
2. Invite family and friends to facility activities and events and encourage them to attend with the residents.
3. Have regularly scheduled family council meetings.
4. Recruit and honor volunteers. Help them feel part of the organization and truly appreciated.
    a. Award special privileges (coffee, use of the copying machine, snacks).
    b. Give volunteers opportunities to meet and socialize with other volunteers and become a part of a group.
    c. Conduct award ceremonies and present certificates of appreciation.
    d. Post the name, picture, contribution, and short biography of the volunteer of the month.
    e. Mention the volunteers' individual contributions in the newsletter.
    f. Publicize what volunteers do for residents each month by tabulating hours and services.
    g. Take and display pictures of volunteers at work.
    h. Remember volunteers on holidays.
5. Mail the monthly newsletter to community organizations and family members.

6. Conduct in-services for family and community members on topics that teach people about long term care facilities such as:
   a. What kind of care to expect in a nursing home.
   b. How to select a nursing home.
   c. Life in a nursing home.
   d. Insurance coverage for nursing home care.
   e. What to do if nursing home care becomes necessary.
   f. Geriatric nursing.
   g. Activities for the impaired elderly.
   h. How to help the nursing home resident.
   i. Visiting tips for nursing home guests.
   j. The elderly and good nutrition.
   k. Providing a safe environment for the elderly.
7. Have community days. Organize an interesting activity, a bar-b-que, or a program, and invite the community. During elections throw a campaign party for the politicians and urge the voters to come and meet them.
8. Encourage the exchange of videos, tapes, and letters among residents and families. Even fill in the blanks letters help keep families involved. These letters can be printed by the facility and residents helped to report their feelings, activities, and up and downs.
9. Notice visitors to the facility. Let them know you are glad they are there.

ORGANIZING THE JOB

So much to do, so little time! Organizing to meet all the requirements relieves stress, makes routine easier, and makes you look good!

1. Tickler files are so effective that any time put into setting them up is a terrific investment in saved time in the future. This is the best way to look and to be organized. Tickler files are good for:

    a. Due dates. Set up tickler files by month for reminders of when to do:

    (1) Quarterly progress notes.

    (2) Care plans.

    (3) Discharge plans.

    (4) Reports for out-of-town families.

    (5) Birthdays, anniversaries, special occasions.

    (6) Medicaid reevaluations.

    b. Specific information. Set up tickler files by subject to keep track of:

    (1) Equipment in residents' possession, such as self-help tools, telephones, communication boards, tape recorders.

    (2) Residents' religion for churches or ministers who want to help or call on parishioners.

    (3) Residents who have no family and need a volunteer support system.

    (4) Veterans, for benefits.

    (5) Who needs help with their social security checks.

    (6) Levels of care.

    (7) Volunteers.

2. Lists. Keep to do lists that can be attached to the appointment calendar. Mark each item with an A, B, or C. The As need to be done today. The Bs can wait a day or so. The Cs may never have to be completed. Cross off the items as they are finished and feel a sense of accomplishment.

3. Calendars. A daily appointment calendar organizes time by letting you know what is scheduled for each day and how much time is available for other duties. Write in all regular meetings and responsibilities at the beginning of each year, such as:

   a. Care plan meetings.

   b. In-service programs.

   c. Staff meetings

   d. Supervisory conferences

   e. Professional conferences and meetings.

   f. Committee meetings

   g. Special programs

   h. Report times

4. Group tasks together. Try to return all telephone calls at one time. Schedule meetings with families on certain days. Set aside time for paper work. Check on residents and make visits using a specific block of times. Always leave some time for whatever might come up.

5. Keep track of time. Learn how much time most projects take so the required amount of time can be scheduled. Mark this in your appointment calendar. Then you will know where the day went and also how to schedule appropriately when the job comes up again.

6. Use small amounts of time. Even when there is not enough time to complete a project, there may be time to organize it. Getting started makes it seem less overwhelming. Using the ten and fifteen minute time spans makes getting through a dreaded task less onerous. Read a report or professional article while waiting. Plan your next day. Write one progress note.

7. Always carry a note-book. Jot down things to remember to do later as the thought comes to you. Make notes of items to include in quarterly progress notes so that time is not wasted with daily charting. Write down your ideas and what you want to discuss with others. Keep your mind clear for the job at hand, not cluttered with trying to remember what has to be done in the future.

8. Keep to the task. There are plenty of distractions, other things to do, and stimuli to capture your attention. Whenever possible complete an unwanted job and then give yourself a reward. This way you have something to look forward to and the unpleasant work is behind you.

9. Handle papers one time. As you go through the mail and other papers that come your way, sort them then. Throw it away, pass it on, file it, or put it aside for thorough reading, answering, or follow-up. If, at the end of a week, you have not had any use for the papers in the follow-up pile, maybe you can throw them away too.

10. Take care of problems. Take notice of difficulties that are brewing and handle them before they become emergencies. Assign the problem to appropriate people, take preventive measures, anticipate the dilemmas that pop up frequently in certain situations and with certain people.

11. Do not let people use you to kill time. Let people know in advance how much time you have. Stand up. Walk to the office door. Make closing statements such as, "Before I leave." Let them know when you will be free to talk, for how long, and where you will meet them.

12. Make decisions. As long as you consider alternatives you cannot move ahead. Take your best shot, make the decision, and get on with the plan.

13. Have an alphabetical filing system. There is no sense in trying to remember everything. It makes good sense to know where to look up things. Keep a file drawer for community resources, special projects, procedures, forms, or anything that might be helpful or come up again. If you can lay your hands on data others want they will be impressed. You can make it look easy.

Go through your files every couple of years to weed out what you have never used or cannot remember why you saved.

14. Determine the important jobs. Some things can be let go indefinitely and no one will notice. Other tasks may seem less of a priority, but need attention because other staff members and the residents will notice. Take care of the parts of your job that involve other people first. Take care of your boss's pet projects. Take care of the tasks that have to be done before other people can do their part. Assist the residents and families who develop high anxiety or need to learn to trust the nursing home staff. Then work on the equally necessary, but less showy elements of your responsibilities.

15. Embrace change. Just because it has always been done that way does not mean it always has to be done the same way. Look for the easier, faster, more efficient way to accomplish a job.

16. Organize your work space. Have what you need handy. Keep paper and pen near the telephone. Have items you use often near or in your desk. Have frequently called telephone numbers posted.

17. Write it down. If you find you are explaining the same thing over and over, such as what the new resident should bring to the facility, or how a referral should be made to social service, write it out. You may still have to explain, but you can use fewer words and back them up with written lists and procedures. If many people need the same information a written message sent or given to all is a time saver.

18. Get a bulletin board for items needed for continuous reference or for reminders.

19. Discipline yourself. If you have a big project that you do not want to do, start on it right away and make yourself spend fifteen to thirty minutes a day on it. In this way the project is underway, gets completed, and you have not had to suffer through it hours on end. A few minutes a day gets it out of the way.

20. Be on time. Minutes lost early in the day cause you to play "catch up" for the rest of the day.

AVOIDING BURN-OUT

We can burn-out in any job. We are never totally satisfied with anything. We get tired of the same things and the same people. Our feelings get hurt. We feel unappreciated. Burn-out is a fact of life.

Burn-out occurs for social workers in long term care facilities for many reasons, a few of which are:

1. Social workers functioning in a medical setting sometimes feel ignored and unrecognized for the contribution they can make to the well-being of the residents and the running of the facility because they do not have a medical focus.
2. Problems tend to repeat themselves. There always are the residents who do not like their roommates, the families who complain and criticize, and the residents who are so disruptive that no one knows what to do about them.
3. There is constant pressure to document and complete paper work to pass numerous critical inspections and licensing processes.
4. The type of people who get into social work are the type who want to be helpful and effect positive change. Most often any change is small, and usually no one person can take credit for the residents' progress because it is a team effort.
5. Even though the residents and staff change over time, the general make-up stays the same. In other words, it is the same people and problems day after day.
6. Once a task is completed it is expected that the due date for completing it another time will arrive again and more quickly than can be imagined.
7. Social service departments are often given the impossible problems to solve.
8. Since nursing homes are medical facilities, social service is sometimes treated as a strange step-child one does not know what to do with and all sorts of miscellaneous projects are

assigned the department, some of which are not appropriate to the discipline.

9. Because social services moves at a different pace and with priorities that are not necessarily the same as the other professionals in the facility they are not always given credit for doing "real work".

In addition to the particular characteristics of social work in a nursing home, social workers may burn-out because of their own traits.

1. Poor social skills. The persons who cannot develop relationships with other staff members will feel isolated and unappreciated. If they cannot get along with others, or if they expect all their social needs to be met in the work place, they will have frustration and disappointment.

2. Cannot say no. The door-mats who cannot define their boundaries and keep letting people dump on them will burn-out from lack of time and skill as they take on more work and unsuitable projects.

    The individuals who cannot turn away any request because they respond to flattery or because they think they are the only ones who can do anything and everything also get caught in the treadmill.

3. Do not differentiate self from job. People whose egos are solely wrapped up in work burn-out because they do not have another self, another identity, other roles in which to find satisfaction.

4. Attracts problems. Employees who get involved with everyone's problems end up with a heavy load. They are there to hear the professional and personal complaints of all the staff members. They end up emotionally seared from others' turmoil, feel they must solve all difficulties, and do not have time to take care of their own lives or do their jobs.

5. Seeks approval. People who cannot tolerate conflict and fear rejection put all their energy into getting approval from others. They will do anything to gain acceptance and are continually looking for signs that people do not like them. Since their

energy is so focused on what other people think, they burn-out in any situation.

6. Expects perfection. Their standards are too high to be realistic, too high to complete the work needing to be done, and higher than their co-workers. They cannot complete a project unless it is perfect, so they fall behind, do not meet their own standards, and are always disappointed in the performance of others. They burn-out.

Prevention of burn-out is the ideal because once burn-out occurs, the damage to the individual's body and mind has been done. At this stage people leave their jobs rather than try to overcome the problems. Leaving the nursing home setting is traumatic because it can give workers a sense of failure, a loss of benefits, and a disappointment that they could not succeed in working in a job they once thought desirable. It is hard for residents to get accustomed to new faces and different styles, and there is always a period of lack of service while new people learn about the residents and the job. It disrupts the team as a new professional has to integrate into the system.

Helpful techniques for preventing burn-out are as follows.

1. No matter what the day has been like, look back over it and note what you have done. Take time to recount all your contacts and recognize your contributions.

2. Pat yourself on the back for your unique contribution as a social worker. See something in the job that only you, in your role, do. Give yourself credit for this.

3. When the work day is over, let it be over. Make a list of what has to be done the next day, what was not completed today, and forget it. Seldom is anything so crucial that it cannot wait. Individuals are not so indispensable that they are needed around the clock. In the morning pick up where you left off. Train yourself to work when at work and to not work when you have time off. That is why you have time off.

4. Realize you cannot do everything. Make referrals. Accept the fact that no one can solve some problems. Do not feel as though you have to be an expert on all things. No one actually expects you to be.

5. Complain, yell, scream if necessary to let off steam. Do this in your car, in front of the mirror, but not to your boss, fellow employees, or the residents.

6. Share your job. Let volunteers, residents' families, and other staff members do their part. Do not be too eager to be helpful. Letting others take responsibility and feel competence is also being helpful.

7. Use humor. When all is tense look at the funny side or tell a joke. Laughter releases tension and changes attitudes.

8. Appreciate other people. Instead of seeing failings, irritating habits, and what others are not doing, change your focus to see what they have done and what you can appreciate about them. Concentrate on their positives. You will see them in a new light. Your feelings will change.

9. Try to remain calm. Ask yourself if it is really worth getting upset, excited, and letting the adrenalin flow. Save your strength. Let others fatigue themselves.

10. Develop a support system. Friends, family, other interests, even pets need to be part of your life. Have people around who will listen and activities that distract and fulfill.

11. Break the routine. Take a new route to work. Schedule your responsibilities in a different order. Use your lunch time for a walk.

12. Decompress. When it all seems too much, take time to think through what brought on the distress. Mentally let go and move on.

13. Find new interest in the work. Learn a new skill. Take on a special project. Make it your business to be an expert on one subject, technique, or resident.

14. Communicate. Know the channels of communication in your facility and keep them open. Use them. When in doubt, ask. When troubled, question. Share what you are doing. Make suggestions. Find out what is going on.

16. Keep current. Do not let the paper work get to be a monster. Stay on top of it. Get it done. Do a little every day and it will not pile up.

RELAXATION

Relaxation is a good stress reliever, enhancing health and feelings of well-being. Even if relaxation did not provide these benefits, the fact that the nursing home residents know that they can control their minds and bodies in this way gives them a needed sense of power.

Relaxation is a technique that must be practiced five to twenty minutes every day. This repetitiveness will enable the residents to learn the skill, master it, and be able to use it as needed.

To learn relaxation the residents must learn:

1. Deep breathing.
2. Concentration.
3. Progressive muscle relaxation.
4. Positive thinking.
5. Imagery.

The procedure is as follows.

1. The residents are seated as comfortably as possible. They hang their heads and close their eyes. They take three deep breaths, imagining that they are breathing in relaxation and breathing out tensions, worries, problems, and aches and pains.
2. The residents are told to concentrate on themselves. All distractions are to be totally disregarded. They are alone in the universe. Nothing can bother or disturb them.
3. Starting at the toes and proceeding slowly to the top of the head the residents are asked to relax each muscle in turn. The residents are told to command their muscles to relax. The muscles respond to the residents' orders.
4. It is suggested that the residents think about their well-being, seeing themselves as a wonderful, worthwhile persons who deserve only the best of everything.

5. With body and mind relaxed and a positive attitude established, the residents are requested to pick out the place they would most like to visit. It is a place where they can be relaxed, continue to feel good about themselves, and have a good time. They imagine themselves there. They know it is a mental trip and they can go to that special place anytime they want to.

6. After a few seconds the residents must say their goodbyes and you count backwards from ten and "return to the room."

REMOTIVATION

Remotivation is an activity in which individuals are given a sense of worth, pleasure, recognition and competency.

Remotivation technique is a simple group method that can be used to reach the impaired residents in a way that gives them a good feeling.

A remotivation group meets regularly, at the same time, in the same place. Although members of the group may come and go, there should be a core group because individuals should be able to look forward to seeing some of the same people. The group leader should not change.

The following structure is suggested for a remotivation group.

1. Greetings.

   Greetings should convey to the group that this is going to be a pleasant experience for everyone, and especially for the leader, who is thrilled to be with them.

   Each group member is greeted individually by name. A personal comment is made to each person. Hand shaking, hugging, or some form of touching is recommended.

2. Structure.

   Residents know what to expect because the same format is followed each meeting. Since the individual is considered a member of this group, changes are made only after discussion in the group. Certain group members will require that the seating be the same each time. These members should be accommodated.

3. Reality.

   The day and date are announced. Any important announcements are made. Are special activities planned? Are there any birthdays, anniversaries, new residents, individuals going home, sicknesses, deaths? Are there any significant changes in the nursing home?

A resident, or the leader, will have the weather report and the major news item of the day. Some item of history is discussed. This may tie in with the news of the day, an impending holiday, or be of general interest. This gives group members an opportunity to explain what they remember of that event, how it affected their lives, or how they prepared for the occurrence. Memories are stimulated. Individuals receive recognition for their contributions. A common bond develops.

4. Activity.

Some simple activity should be planned. No particular skill need be required. It should be a game of chance where there is one winner who receives the distinct honor of being the victor of the day. You may have the group roll dice, pull papers, pick numbers, or bounce a ball a certain number of times. The joy of competition and the anticipation of winning gives the game its sharp edge.

5. A challenge.

A simple, short quiz is suggested. There are any number in publications for the elderly. A few questions helps the members to think and gives them pleasure when they come up with the correct answer.

A short joke is also fun and enlivening. Residents may want to contribute a joke of their own. A good laugh is not only fun, but healthy.

6. Refreshments.

As members of the group they share in a special treat. They are offered something to eat or drink. The serving is personal and individualized. The comfort of each is stressed. When members are ready to leave they should be given assistance to their destination.

RESOCIALIZATION

Resocialization is a progressive program that begins where the residents are in their social skills and capitalizes on their interests and abilities.

The steps are as follows.

1. Introduce resident to one other resident. Make arrangements for them to see each other regularly.
2. Introduce the residents to another resident after they know the first one well enough to incorporate another person into their lives.
3. Continue individual introductions until there are enough residents who know each other for a small group of three to four.
4. Show the residents pictures of their new friends and reward them when they correctly identify them.
5. Have frequent time-limited get-togethers for this new group. Make them pleasant and interesting. Reward interaction with approval and praise.
6. Arrange for the residents to attend an activity related to their interests.
7. Make arrangements for the individuals to attend this activity (sports event, musical program, shopping, a drive, play, movie) with new acquaintances.
8. Invite residents and new acquaintances to a group event in the nursing home such as a birthday party.
9. Reinstitute resocialization program at any level whenever needed.

This program should enable the residents to focus on others rather than self.

NURSING HOME VISITING TIPS

Visits are encouraged from anyone in the community and are meaningful to the nursing home residents. This list of visiting suggestions may be helpful to you as you visit your friend or relative.

1. Go for a ride. Residents sometimes have little opportunity to see how the community has changed, to view the scenery, or to see their previous home. Such an outing brings back memories and enlarges the world of the nursing home residents.

2. Visitors are invited to participate in any of the activities. A planned activity is something to do together and can serve to encourage inactive residents to find pleasure in a regularly scheduled event. Check the activity calendar to choose exercises, crafts, parties, or whatever appeals to you.

3. Bring your own activity. What did your friend or relative like to do before placement in the nursing home? Go for a walk. Play cards. Throw a ball. Listen to a ball game. Watch a favorite TV show together. Have a picnic on the patio. You will have your own ideas. Bring in a pet to play with and discuss.

4. Celebrate a special event. A party is always special and fun. Your friend or relative can be the "Guest of Honor" for whatever occasion you wish to celebrate.

5. Come for lunch. Plan your visit around a meal time and socialize while eating.

6. Bring in pictures. Ask your loved ones to identify and explain old pictures. Bring them up-to-date by showing and telling the residents about newer family members. Show vacation pictures too!

7. Reminisce. The old remember what it was like to be young. Ask about life in the "old days" and learn something about your roots. Obtain a "Grandparents" book from your local book store and record the answers for the generations to come.

8. Share your talents. Are you learning something new? Practice your Spanish, your musical instrument, or your handiwork with your friends or relatives and see if they can notice your improvement from one visit to the next.

9. Show and tell. What is new in your life? Are you excited about a new car, a new set of tools or dishes, or a new outfit? Bring it along and show it off.

10. Help. Perhaps your loved ones need their clothes and belongings marked with their identification. Go through the closets and drawers, labeling where each item is kept. Sometimes identifying pictures are more helpful than words.

11. Create a feeling. We all respond and do better when we feel approval and caring. Provide an atmosphere of pleasant concern and security. Find some way to give a compliment or something to appreciate.

12. Touch. We all need physical contact with other human beings. Use your visiting opportunity to hold your loved one's hand. Give encouraging and affectionate pats and a hug.

13. Give attention. Individual attention is a wonderful thing. Make sure your friends or relatives know that they have your attention. Look at them when they speak and as you talk to them. They need to feel your undivided attention.

14. Be positive. Try to distract complaining residents by bringing up a cheerful event, telling a joke, or recalling a pleasant incident. Do not get caught up in the negative aspects of living. Make your visit a happy event. Concentrate on feeling positive about your loved one's situation. Do not allow yourself to get bogged down in feelings of guilt, resentment, or self-blaming. This is not helpful to you or the residents.

15. Identify yourself. Sometimes it may be necessary to remind your friends or relatives of your name and relationship to them.

16. Adhere to safety rules. Because of the danger of fire, smoking is allowed only in the activity and dining rooms. Help us protect your loved ones by retaining possession of cigarettes and matches.

17. Bring a special treat. Sharing favorite foods is appreciated. But also share our concern for cleanliness and contamination. All foods must be contained in a sealed plastic or metal container if it is to be kept in the resident's room. Label all items with the resident's name. Make sure you check first with the nurse or dietician for any possible dietary restrictions.

18. Participate. The Resident Council is an important part of the nursing home administration. Relatives and friends are invited to attend the Advisory Committee meetings and hear the concerns and the residents' suggested solutions.

19. Toast your relationship. If social drinking is allowed by the resident's physician, feel free to enjoy a cocktail together.

INDEX

A

Abusive	.45
Active listening	.94
Adjustment	.42
Aggressive	.58
Aging process, do not accept	.49
Agitated	.54
Altered self-image	.38
Alzheimer's disease	.56
Anger	.32
Angry	.58
Anticipate needs	95, 59
Anxiety	.54
Appreciate other people	108
Apprehensive	.51
Avoiding burnout	105

B

Bedridden	.62
Behavior modification	38, 95
Boredom	.52
Break the routine	108
Burn-out	105

C

Cancer	.35
Care plan	.3, 4, 24
Care plan meetings	. 5
Choices	.49
Combative	.58
Communicate	108
Communication, non-verbal	.90
Community resources	.17
Compensated	.48
Complains about physical health	.66
Complains of unhappiness	.30
Confrontive	.59
Cries frequently	.30
Criticizes	.34
Current functioning	.11

D

Death of a loved one	.41
Decompress	108
Delusion	.65
Demanding	.51
Demonstrate the wanted behavior	.97
Denial	.33
Dependent	59, 60
Desire to die	.37
Deteriorates	.49
Diagnosis, does not accept	.32
Discharge	.10
Discharge limitations	.19
Discharge plan	.10, 13, 17
Discipline yourself	104
Disoriented	45, 66
Distraction	64, 91

E

Evaluate 24
Explosive 58
Express self verbally, cannot 50

F

Family council meeting 50
Family unhappy with resident's care 44
Family visits 43
Fear of bath 62
Fear of loss of ability 48
Fearful of dying .32
Fears 32
Feeding self, difficulty 53
Feeling of uselessness 39
Find new interest in the work 108
Friends, difficulty making 66
Funds 32

G

Gets lost 56
Grief 30
Guidance, give non-threatening 93

H

Hallucinations 67
Hearing, loss of 46
Help residents regain their composure 93
Helpless 61

Hides dirty laundry 46
Hope 36
Hopeless 30
Hugs 51
Hyperventilates 54

I

Incontinent 46
Independent 60
Inservices, conduct for family 100
Invite family 99
Involve residents in doing 92
Isolate 50

K

Keep current 108

L

"Living Will" 37
Lonely 50
Looks for people no longer part of her life 56
Loss 48

M

Malnourished 63
Manipulates 61, 59
Meaningful task 39
Model 36

Modeled 52
Modeling behavior 97
Mood swings 57
Motivation, lack of 48

N

No interest in activities 31
Non-verbal 50, 63

O

Organize work space 104
Organizing the job 101

P

Pain 35
Palpitations 54
Parkinson's disease 53
Participation 92
Pat yourself on the back 107
Pets 52
Placement on discharge 18
Positive reinforcement 62
Praise 40
Prognosis, family does not accept 34
Prognosis, not accepting the 30
Progress note 83

Q

Quarterly progress notes .83

R

Re-direct 93
Reality orientation 57, 87
Realize you cannot do everything 107
Reassurance 54, 55, 91
Recognition 59
Recruit and honor volunteers 99
Referral log 21
Refocusing 48
Refuses activities 35
Refuses medication 37
Refuses to eat 37
Refuses to get out of bed 31
Refuses to see doctor .63
Refusing food 30
Refusing to see family 34
Relaxation 42, 109
Reminisce 30, 37, 98
Remotivation 57, 111
Resocialization 42, 51, 113
Restorative techniques 90

S

Sees no reason to live .31
Self-esteem 39
Self-esteem Enhancement 89
Share your job 108
Short attention span .64
Sleeplessness 42

Smoking, unsafe 47
Social history 11
Social service assessment 9
Social service Needs 12
Strengths 83
Stroke 38
Suicidal 40
Support system, develop a 108
Supportive 93
Suspicious 58

T

Team 3
Terminally ill 30
Time, keep track of 102
Tremors 53
Try to remain calm 108

U

Unresponsive 62
Use humor 108
Useless 38

V

Validation 88
Validation approach .57
Verbally abusive 57, 58
Vision, loss of 46
Visiting tips 114
Volunteers 99

W

Walk, inability to 38
Wanders 66
Wants to die 37
Whines 66
Will not get out of bed .37
Withdrawing 35
Withdrawing from social contacts 30
Worried 32
Write it down 104

Y

Yells 62

M & H PUBLISHING CO. INC.,
P.O. Box 268, La Grange, Texas, 78945-0268

NUM.	QUAN.	DESCRIPTION	PRICE	COST
101	_____	New Health Care Planning For Nurses In Long Term Care	14.45	_____
102	_____	Texas Policies And Procedures Manual	75.00	_____
103	_____	Nursing Procedures Manual	33.50	_____
104	_____	Care Plans That Work	54.45	_____
105	_____	National Policies And Procedures	49.95	_____
106	_____	Activity Care Plans For Long Term Care Facilities—Revised	19.95	_____
108	_____	Writing Health Care Plans, A Handbook For Food Serv. Super.	13.95	_____
109	_____	The Idea Book For Activity Programs	45.95	_____
B110	_____	Introduction To Health Care Administration	89.00	_____
111	_____	Dietary Policies And Procedures	29.50	_____
112	_____	Activity And Volunteer Service Policies And Procedures	34.95	_____
C113	_____	A Programmed Manual For Nursing Home Administrator Exam.	27.50	_____
114	_____	Revised Social Service Care Plans For Nursing Homes	14.95	_____
115	_____	Inservice Manual Continuing Educ. Prog. For Long Term C.	31.95	_____
B117	_____	Cost Management For Long Term Care Facilities	49.95	_____
B118	_____	A Handbook For Health Records In Long-term Care	48.85	_____
119	_____	The Nursing Home And The Resident's Relatives	14.95	_____
121	_____	Wake Up! A Sensory Stimulation Program For Nurs. Home Res.	9.95	_____
B122	_____	The Review Manual For The National Nurs. Home Admin. Exam.	25.95	_____
B123	_____	Criteria For Preceptors Of Administrators-in-training Prog.	55.00	_____
D127	_____	Decubitus Ulcers - Resource Manual And Training Guide	38.95	_____
128	_____	Infection Control	8.95	_____
129	_____	Enhancing The Self Esteem Of The Nursing Home Resident	9.95	_____
130	_____	When The Nursing Home Is The Only Choice	5.95	_____
131	_____	Cycle Menus I With Diet Modifications And Selected Recipes	49.95	_____
C132	_____	Pre-exam For Nursing Home Administrator Examinees	7.50	_____
135	_____	Enteral Feedings In The Nursing Home	10.95	_____
136	_____	Mental Health Problems And The Nursing Home Resident	14.95	_____
B137	_____	Maintenance Management For Health Care Facilities	39.95	_____
138	_____	Favorite Hymns & Gospel Songs	6.95	_____
139	_____	Communicable Diseases Policies and Procedures	23.95	_____
E140	_____	The Internal Audit System	169.00	_____
141	_____	Rehabilitative and Restorative Nursing In The LTC Facility	10.95	_____
142	_____	Training Program for Nurse Aides in the Long Term Care Facility	39.95	_____
F143	_____	Keep Minds Alert I	11.95	_____
F144	_____	Let's Play the Date II	14.95	_____
G145	_____	Realistic Alzheimers Activities	7.95	_____
G146	_____	Memory Sharing	8.95	_____
G147	_____	Fun For Everyone	16.95	_____
G148	_____	Where Does Your Garden Grow?	10.95	_____
G149	_____	Nature Crafts For Every Season	6.95	_____
G150	_____	Creating With Ease	21.95	_____
F151	_____	Now & Then III	5.95	_____
F152	_____	Date'n Game IV	17.95	_____
G154	_____	Activities Digest	21.95	_____
G155	_____	Bible Studies for Senior Citizens	9.95	_____

Continued on the next Page—Please complete the order form on the next page

CONTINUED FROM PREVIOUS PAGE

M & H PUBLISHING CO. INC.

P.O. Box 268, La Grange, Texas, 78945-0268

NUM.	QUAN.	DESCRIPTION	PRICE	COST
157	_____	Who's In Charge Here? A Guidebook for the LTC Charge Nurse	10.95	_____
158	_____	Preparation for Skilled Conditions of Participation	29.95	_____
159	_____	The Restorative Approach for Nursing Home Social Workers	10.95	_____
H161	_____	VHS Tape "Choking: Prevention and Intervention" (23 minutes)	89.00	_____
~~H162~~	_____	~~VHS Tape "I Have Rights Too" (25 minutes)~~	~~89.00~~	_____
H163	_____	VHS Tape "Infection Control - Part 1: The Nursing Aspect" (30 minutes)	89.00	_____
H164	_____	VHS Tape "Confidentiality of Patient Information" (20 minutes)	89.00	_____
H165	_____	VHS Tape "Body Mechanics: Moving and Lifting the Resident" (25 minutes)	89.00	_____
B166	_____	Public Relations Can Be Fun and Easy	14.95	_____
J167	_____	Professional 365 Day Planning Calendar	9.95	_____
K168	_____	The Activity Director's Bag of Tricks	10.95	_____
K169	_____	The Activity Director's Treasure Chest	7.95	_____
L170	_____	This and That	11.95	_____
L171	_____	More This and That	11.95	_____
M172	_____	Failure-Free Activities for the Alzheimer's Patient	10.95	_____
M173	_____	Reminiscence — Uncovering a lifetime of memories	11.95	_____
174	_____	Cycle Menus II	49.95	_____
175	_____	A Personal Orientation Manual	18.95	_____
176	_____	Nursing Management in the 90's	19.95	_____
B177	_____	Songs to Remember Vol I	11.95	_____
B178	_____	Songs to Remember Vol II	11.95	_____
179	_____	Developing and Managing a N.H. Volunteer Program	14.95	_____
181	_____	Social Service Policies and Procedures for LTC Facilities	24.95	_____
182	_____	Alzheimer's Disease: Activities that Work	14.95	_____
F183	_____	ABC Games	7.95	_____
184	_____	Generic Person Stamp	19.95	_____
N17601	_____	Quality Assurance Form (8 1/2 x 11; 100 per pad)	5.59	_____
N17625	_____	Accident Report Form (8 1/2 x 11; 100 per pad)	5.59	_____
N17645	_____	Care Plan Form (2 sides 8 1/2 x 11; 100 per pad)	6.99	_____
185	_____	Quality Assurance with Care Planning	85.00	_____
B186	_____	Activities for the Mind	39.95	_____
P187	_____	Cassette Tape; Alzheimers Disease: Activities that Work	6.95	_____
F189	_____	Moments from the Bible	10.95	_____

NOTE: Prices Subject to Change Without Notice!

POSTAGE AND HANDLING (1 item $2.50, 2 items $4.00, 3 items $5.00, 4 or more items $6.00) _____

SUB-TOTAL _____

Texas Residents add SALES TAX _____

TOTAL _____

NAME OF FACILITY

NAME   TITLE

ADDRESS

CITY   STATE   ZIP CODE

For Orders — Call 1-800-521-9950